Copyright 2020 by Kevin Lewis -All rights reserved.

No part of this book may be reproduced or transmitted in any form or by any means, electronic or mechanical, including photocopying and recording, or by any information storage and retrieval system, without permission in writing from the publisher. This is a work of fiction. Names, places, characters and incidents are either the product of the author's imagination or are used fictitiously, and any resemblance to any actual persons, living or dead, organizations, events or locales is entirely coincidental. The unauthorized reproduction or distribution of this copyrighted work is ilegal.

Disclaimer Notice:

Please note the information contained within this document is for educational and entertainment purposes only. All effort has been executed to present accurate, up to date, reliable, complete information. No warranties of any kind are declared or implied. Readers acknowledge that the author is not engaged in the rendering of legal, financial, medical, or professional advice. The content within this book has been derived from various sources. Please consult a licensed professional before attempting any techniques outlined in this book.

By reading this document, the reader agrees that under no circumstances is the author responsible for any losses, direct or indirect, that are incurred as a result of the use of the information contained within this document, including, but not limited to, errors, omissions, or inaccuracies.

CONTENTS

- Introduction 6
- Chapter 1: Keto details 7
  - Benefits of keto diet 7
  - Keto Plate (What should consist on the plate of a keto follower) 7
  - What to eat 7
  - Getting started tips 10
- Chapter 2: Breakfast 12
  - Breakfast Cheesy Sausage 12
  - Cauliflower Toast with Avocado 12
  - Keto Avocado Toast 12
  - Chocolate Chip Waffles 12
  - Egg Crepes with Avocados 13
  - Ham and Cheese Pockets 13
  - Clementine and Pistachio Ricotta 13
  - Avo-Tacos 14
  - The Asian Chickpea Pancake 14
  - Overnight Oat Bowl 14
  - Coconut Crepes 15
  - Matcha Avocado Pancakes 15
  - Low-Carb Breakfast "Couscous" 15
  - Gingerbread-Spiced Breakfast Smoothie 15
  - Vegan Breakfast Muffins 16
  - Vegan Breakfast Biscuits 16
  - Vegan Breakfast Sausages 16
  - Quick Breakfast Yogurt 16
  - Spiced Tofu and Broccoli Scramble 17
  - Meat-Free Breakfast Chili 17
  - Vegan Southwestern Breakfast 17
  - Egg Roll Bowl 18
  - Keto Breakfast Porridge 18
  - Keto Choco "Oats" 18
  - Banana Hazelnut Waffles 18
  - Vegan Breakfast Skillet 19
  - Vegan Breakfast Hash 19
  - Tiramisu Chia Pudding 19
  - Tofu and Spinach Frittata 19
  - Fat-Bomb Frappuccino 20
- Chapter 3: Soups & Salads 21
  - Instant Pot Beans & Ham Soup 21
  - Truffle Parmesan Salad 21
  - Cashew Siam Salad 21
  - Kelp noodle salad 22
  - Tasty Green Salad 22
  - Asparagus and Artichoke Salad 22
  - Spicy Satay Tofu Salad 23
  - Thai Chicken Coconut Soup 23
  - Ham And Green Bean Soup 24
  - Superfood Soup 24
  - Avgolemono Soup 25
  - Barbecue Chicken Pizza Soup 25
  - Spicy Cauliflower Soup 25
  - Vegan Cream Of Broccoli Soup 26
  - Cream Of Mushroom Soup 26
  - Cream Of Tomato Soup 27
  - Yellow-beet salad with anchovies 27
  - Vegan Cream Of Broccoli Soup 27
  - Cream Of Mushroom Soup 27
  - Spinach & Cauliflower Soup 28
  - Oriental red cabbage salad 28
  - Broccoli salad with fresh dill 29
  - Zucchini salad with eggs 29
  - Low-carb fried kale and broccoli salad. 29
  - Mixed cabbage coleslaw 30
  - Seafood salad with avocado 30
  - Jalapeno Bacon Cheddar Soup 30
  - Chicken Lime Soup 31
  - Jalapeno Pepper Soup 31
  - Chicken Chili Soup 32
- Chapter 4: Vegetables & Side Dishes 33
  - Easy Cheesy Artichokes 33
  - Chinese Bok Choy 33
  - Green Cabbage with Bacon 33
  - Warm Broccoli Salad Bowl 34
  - Creamed Spinach with Cheese 34
  - Cheesy Spinach 34
  - Creamy Brussels Sprout 35
  - Broccoli Stir Fry 35
  - Spicy Mushrooms 35
  - Cauliflower Mash 36
  - Cauliflower Soufflé 36
  - Garbanzo and Spinach Beans 36
  - Delicious Garlic Tomatoes 37
  - Mashed Celeriac 37
  - Apple Slices 37
  - Cashew Sauce 37
  - Japanese Cabbage Dish 38
  - Almond Buttery Green Cabbage 38
  - Brussels and Pistachios 38
  - Brussels's Fever 39
  - Garlic and Kale Platter 39
  - Acorn Squash with Mango Chutney 39
  - Honey and Coconut Porridge 39
  - Maple Glazed Carrots 40

- Ginger and Orange "Beets" 40
- Baby Potatoes 40
- Cauliflower Cakes 40
- Coconut and Cauliflower Rice with Chili ... 41
- Fried Apple 41
- Spaghetti Squash 41
- Garlic and Mushroom Crunch 41
- Pepper Jack Cauliflower 42
- The Brussels Platter 42
- Southern Salad 42
- Kale and Carrot with Tahini Dressing 42
- Crispy Kale 43
- Summertime Veggies 43
- Caramelized Onion 43
- Kidney Beans and Cilantro 43
- Broccoli Crunchies 44
- Buffalo Cashews 44
- A Green Bean Mixture 44
- Cauliflower and Mushroom Risotto 45
- Zucchini Boats 45
- Roasted Onions and Green Beans 45
- Green Bean Roast 45
- Almond and Blistered Beans 46
- Tomato Platter 46
- Lemony Sprouts 46
- Cauliflower Rice 47

Chapter 5: Main Dishes 48
- Stuffed Zucchini 48
- Avocado Fries 48
- Mushroom Zoodle Pasta 49
- Quick Veggie Protein Bowl 49
- Vizza 49
- Tofu Cheese Nuggets & Zucchini Fries ... 50
- Avocado Spring Rolls 51
- Cauliflower Curry Soup 51
- Crispy Tofu Burgers 52
- Baked Chicken Fajitas 52
- Baked Chicken Wings 53
- Chicken with Spinach Broccoli 53
- Delicious Bacon Chicken 53
- Mexican Chicken 53
- Beef Casserole 54
- Mexican Beef with Zucchini 54
- Mexican Beef 54
- Asian Beef Stew 55
- Beef Roast 55
- Almond Cinnamon Beef Meatballs 55
- Creamy Beef Stroganoff 56
- Buttery Lamb Chops 56
- Lemon Herb Lamb Chops 56
- Fennel Grill Pork Chops 57
- Herb Pork Roast 57
- Asian Pork Hock 57
- Parmesan Meatballs 58
- Beef Shawarma 58
- Shrimp and Broccoli 58
- Baked Salmon 58
- Buttery Shrimp 59
- Avocado Shrimp Salad 59
- Shrimp and Garlic 59
- Salmon Patties 59
- Tuna Salad 60
- Shrimp Scampi 60
- Grilled Salmon 60
- Salmon with Sauce 60
- Parmesan Salmon 61
- Shrimp Stir Fry 61
- Zucchini Eggplant with Cheese 61
- Turnips Mashed 61
- Coconut Cauliflower Rice 62
- Parmesan Zucchini Chips 62
- Olive Cheese Omelet 62
- Cheese Almond Pancakes 62
- Cauliflower Frittata 63
- Basil Tomato Frittata 63
- Chia Spinach Pancakes 63
- Feta Kale Frittata 63
- Protein Muffins 64

Chapter 6: Breads & Rolls 65
- Low-carb dinner rolls 65
- Low-carb clover rolls 65
- Keto bread rolls 65
- Keto coconut bread rolls 66
- Low carb bread rolls (without eggs) 66
- Avocado Mug Bread 67
- Sausage bread 67
- Cheese sausage bread 67
- Hazelnut honey bread 67
- Coconut milk bread 68
- Egg bread 68
- Simple keto bread 69
- Multi-grain bread 69
- Toast bread 70
- Walnut bread 70
- Bulgur bread 70
- Italian blue cheese bread 71
- German bread linz 71

- Apple bread with horseradish and pistachios 71
- Honey bread with cream and coconut milk 71
- Milk almond bread 72
- Almond bread with a delicate crust 72
- Rice bread 72
- Rice bread with soy sauce 73
- Cumin bread 73

Chapter 7: Appetizers & Beverages 74
- Iced Keto Coffee 74
- Jicama Fries 74
- Keto Mocha 74
- Keto Turkish Coffee 74
- Keto Ice Cream Coffee mix 75
- Butter Coffee 75
- Thai Iced Tea 75
- Vanilla Custard 75
- Vanilla Pana Cotta 75
- Creamy Cinnamon Coffee 76
- Chia Seed Pudding 76
- Tasty Chicken Egg Rolls 76
- Avocado Gazpacho 77
- Spinach Chips 77
- Parsley Dip 77
- Kale Muffins 77
- Cream Cheese Spread 77
- Beef Muffins 78
- Herbs Spread 78
- Thyme Leek Snack Bowls 78
- Cilantro and Leeks Dip 78
- Shrimp Bowls 78
- Cheddar Cauliflower Bites 79
- Turmeric Dip 79
- Tomato Dip 79

Chapter 8: Desserts 80
- Cheesecake Bites 80
- Chocolate Chip Balls 80
- Coconut Bars 80
- Frozen Yogurt 80
- Key Lime Pie 81
- Raspberry Ice Cream 81
- Yogurt Popsicles 81
- Vanilla Berry Mug Cake 81
- Pumpkin Spice Mug Cake 82
- Lemon Coconut Cake 82
- No Bake Coconut Bars 83
- Peanut Butter Bars 83
- Coconut Chocolate Bars 84
- Chocolate Fudge Bars 84
- Granola Bars 85
- Lemon Bars 85
- Chocolate Cake 85
- Cinnamon & Nutmeg Cake 86
- Coffee Cake 87
- Cream & Berries Cake 87
- Chocolate Bonbons 88
- Chocolate Coconut Bites 88
- Chocolate Covered Almonds 89
- Almond Joy 89
- Candy Dots 89
- Lemon Cheesecake Mousse 89
- English Custard 90
- Pumpkin Cheesecake Mousse 90
- Cheesecake Pudding 90
- Coconut Lemon Custard Pie 91

Chapter 9: Cookies & Candy 92
- Fifth Avenue Candy 92
- Chocolate Chip Cookies 92
- Chocolate Coconut Cookies 92
- Coconut No-Bake Cookies 93
- Cream Cheese Cookies 93
- Ginger Snap Cookies 93
- Nut Butter Cookies 93
- Orange Walnut Cookies 94
- Boston Baked Beans Candy 94
- Fresh Breath Mints 94
- Peanut Brittle 94
- Crystal Candy Skewers 95
- Pecan Brittle Squares 95
- Brittle Butterscotch Candy 95
- Pecan Candies 96
- Bourbon Candy Balls 96
- Mixed Nuts Choco Candy Clusters 97
- Crispy Cookies 97
- Nutty Cookies 97
- Snickerdoodle Cookies 98

Chapter 10: Smoothies 99
- Blueberry and Soy Smoothie 99
- Blueberry Avocado Smoothie 99
- Blackberry Smoothie 99
- Berry Acai Smoothie 99
- Choco-Coco Milk Shake 99
- Nutty Choco Milk Shake 100
- Choco Milk Smoothie 100
- Creamy Choco Shake 100
- Baby Kale and Yogurt Smoothie 100
- Nutty Arugula Yogurt Smoothie 100

- Hazelnut-Lettuce Yogurt Shake 100
- Garden Greens & Yogurt Shake 101
- Ginger-Spiced Coconut-Milk Shake 101
- Strawberry Coconut Shake...................... 101
- Hazelnut and Coconut Shake.................. 101
- Cardamom-Cinnamon Spiced Coco-Latte 101
- Hazelnut-Mocha Shake 102
- Fruity Morning Smoothie......................... 102
- Creamy Wake-Me-Up Smoothie 102
- Chocolate-Coconut Shake 102

Chapter 11: This & That.................................... 103
- Almond Pumpkin Pudding 103
- Chocolate Avocado Pudding 103
- Butter Tossed Asparagus.......................... 103
- Caramelized Onions 103
- Curry Mayonnaise 104
- Green Tahini 104
- Cheesy Fondue.. 104
- Green Bean Fries 104
- Celery and Almond Butter 105
- Salted Macadamias 105
- Almond Butter Fat Bombs 105
- Tahini Sauce.. 105
- Baked Brie 106
- Spicy Mayo 106
- Raspberry Chia Pudding........................... 106
- Raspberry Chocolate Fudge 106
- Strawberry Chia Pudding Popsicles 107
- Red Pepper Cod.. 107
- Beef Stew 107
- Fish Tacos 108

Appendix : Recipes Index 109

Introduction

Thank you for choosing this book.

Many health advocates claim that a healthy diet must consist of a balance of healthy fats, Carbs, and protein. Although fats are almost always part of this equation, it still holds a bad reputation as causing weight gain due to its high-calorie content and the fact that it is still associated – albeit misguidedly – with what causes fat to accumulate in the blood vessels and on the body. As a result, it is often said that fat should be limited to very small amounts in a person's diet, leaving only room for mostly protein and Carbs instead. In truth, Carbs and fats should switch places in this equation.

When you replace the Carbs in your diet with healthy fats, and also keep the amount of Carbs you eat to a minimum, a process occurs that results in your metabolism responding by behaving as it would if you were fasting (abstaining from foods for a long period of time) or if you had just exercised for a prolonged period.

This book contains information on keto diet and its various benefits. There are also 300 keto recipes that you can easily prepare at home.

Thanks for choosing this book. Enjoy reading!

Chapter 1: Keto details

Benefits of keto diet

Improves Brain function
Keto diet is low carb diet which will decrease your blood glucose and insulin level. During the fat breaking process, fatty acids are released and your liver produces ketones from fatty acids. These ketones full fill 70 percent of your brain energy needs. Scientific research and study prove that a keto diet is very effective to treat a brain-related disease like epilepsy, Alzheimer's and Parkinson's disease.

Weight loss
Compare to another diet ketogenic diet is very effective on weight loss. It gives you long term weight loss benefits. Our bodies use glucose for energy as a primary source. When on the keto diet, instead of your body breaking down glucose, it will break down the fats. When you consume a moderate amount of protein during keto diet means it doesn't feel you a hungry compared to another diet. This will reduce your body weight rapidly and you will get long term weight loss benefits during a ketogenic diet.

Maintains Blood sugar level
Basically keto diet is low carb diet due to this it helps to reduce your blood sugar level and insulin level. One of the scientific research and study proves that a keto diet is very effective in treating type-2 diabetes. To transport into your body cells glucose needs insulin and also increase insulin sensitivity. On the other side, ketones don't need insulin to transport into a body cell. Due to this your blood sugar level are maintain and stable throughout the day.

Increase HDL cholesterol and Improve LDL cholesterol level
Keto diet is low carb and high-fat diet helps to increase good HDL (High-density lipoprotein) cholesterol level in blood. Smaller bad LDL particles are leads to you towards heart disease. Low carb diet helps to increase the size of bad LDL particles. Which help to reduce the number of total LDL particles in the bloodstream. Lowering carb intake helps to improve your heart function and reduce the risk of heart disease.

Works on various disease
While you are on a keto diet your body uses ketones for energy. Ketones are antioxidant and anti-inflammatory properties. It helps to treat some brain conditions like Alzheimer's, Parkinson's and epilepsy. It is also effective for type-2 diabetes, cancer, and heart-related disease.

Keto Plate (What should consist on the plate of a keto follower)

Beef, Pork, Lamb, Chicken, Turkey, Organ meats, Salmon, Mackerel, Sardines, Herring, Cod, Seafood, Butter, Cream, Sour Cream, Soft/Hard Cheese, Greek/Bulgarian Yogurt, Regular Yogurt (sugar-free), Butter, Coconut oil, Olive oil, Ghee, Chicken fat, Avocados, Mayonnaise, High-fat sauces, Green leafy veggies, Broccoli/Cabbage, Brussels sprouts, Asparagus, Zucchini, Eggplant, Olives Mushrooms, Cucumber, Lettuce, Avocado, Onions & Garlic, Soy Sauce, Lemon and lime juice Sriracha Sauce, Homemade mayo, Dijon mustard Wholegrain mustard, Hot sauces, Erythritol, Stevia, Splenda, Brand-name sugar replacements, Monk Fruit Sugar & Syrup, Salad dressings (homemade only), Champagne (sugar-free),
Red or white wine Whiskey/Brandy, Tequila Vodka Soda, Dry Martini

What to eat

Below is a list you should include on your menu:

Vegetables
You will eat tons of vegetables on the keto diet. However, you should be more attentive about the kinds of vegetables you consume. Eat vegetables high in nutrients and low in Carbs. Organic vegetables are the best, as they contain fewer chemicals and pesticides. The greatest advantage for eating non-starchy vegetables is that they do not raise your blood glucose levels, which

would throw your ketosis off balance. Non-starchy vegetables can also help you lose weight by reducing your appetite because they are loaded with fiber.

Here is a short list of some of the best vegetables to eat on the ketogenic diet:

Lettuce
Lettuce is the best vegetable for a ketogenic lifestyle. Lettuce contains few Carbsand is a great source of potassium, protein, fiber, and energy.

Broccoli
Broccoli is healthy and delicious and rich in nutrients, fiber, calcium, protein, and potassium.

Spinach
Spinach is one of the best vegetables rich in potassium, proteins, and iron. Spinach is also delicious and can be used for salads, stuffing, side dishes, and much more.

Cauliflower
Cauliflower is an excellent source of choline, dietary fiber, omega-3 fatty acids, phosphorus, biotin, vitamins B1, B2, and B3. You can use cauliflower to prepare rice, pizza crusts, hummus, and breadsticks.

Tomatoes
Tomatoes carry many positive health benefits and are a great source of vitamin A, C, and K. Including these vitamins, tomatoes are high in potassium, which can reduce blood pressure levels and decrease stroke risks. When you roast tomatoes with olive oil, you can enhance the lycopene content, boosting its effects. It can also protect heart health and reduce the risk of cancer.

Avocados
Avocados are rich in omega oils. Avocados can be consumed in salads or mixed with other ingredients such as yogurt and nuts. They are high in potassium and fiber and are great for your metabolism and heart. Most grocery stores will sell them in a semi-ripened condition, so you can keep them for up to a week as they ripen. Avocados also have high oil content and minerals, which reduce your appetite and provide nutrients all around for your body.

Asparagus
Asparagus is a great source of minerals and vitamins, including vitamin A, C, and K. Studies have shown that asparagus can help cope with anxiety and protect mental health. Consider eating roasted asparagus for dinner or add raw asparagus in your salads.

Mushrooms
Mushrooms contain strong anti-inflammatory properties, which can improve inflammation for those who have metabolic problems. Mushrooms are also packed with copper, potassium, protein, and selenium. It is also a great source of phosphorus, niacin, pantothenic acid, and zinc, especially if you cook them until brown.

Zucchini
Zucchini is low-carb vegetable and a great source of vitamin A, magnesium, potassium, copper, phosphorus, and folate. Zucchini is also high in omega-3 fatty acids, protein, zinc, and niacin. If you include zucchini in your diet, it can lead to an optimal healthy lifestyle.

Bell Peppers
Bell peppers are nutritious and packed with fiber and vitamins. Bell peppers also contain anti-inflammatory properties that are useful on the ketogenic diet.

Proteins
Following a ketogenic diet requires you to find a source of protein. Proteins consist of amino acids, which are essential nutrients for your body and brain. You need to consume protein, as it is your primary fuel source on this diet. Here are some things you might consider adding to your plate:

Meat and Poultry

Any kind of meat can be used for the ketogenic diet, especially if they are high in fat. Always choose meat from grass-fed and wild animal sources. Avoid hot dogs and sausages, and meat covered with starch or processed sauces.

Fish

Fish is another great source of protein. As with meat and poultry, always choose organic and wild fish caught naturally. Examples of good fish include salmon, trout, tuna, shrimp, cod, lobster, and catfish.

Eggs

Eggs are an incredible source of protein and contain low carbs, especially the egg yolk.

Fats and Oils

Since you will need to burn fat for energy, include fats and oils in your diet. Instead of vegetable oil, go for olive oil, coconut oil, avocado oil, and ghee.

Also, buy oils that are rich in polyunsaturated fats and have a low smoke level; these oils will retain their fatty acids. Such oils include walnut oil, flax oil, hemp seed oil, and grape seed oil.

Dairy Products

For a ketogenic diet, consider consuming raw and organic dairy products. You can use cheeses and creams to prepare ketogenic meals. Examples of the best dairy products to include in your diet are mozzarella cheese, cheddar cheese, parmesan cheese, cottage cheese, sour cream, cream cheese, heavy whipping cream, and Greek yogurt.

Nuts and Seeds

Nuts contain healthy fats and nutrients such as vitamin E. When choosing nuts, purchase roasted nuts because they already have their anti-nutrients discarded. Best nuts and seeds for this diet include walnuts, almonds, and macadamias. They are low in calories and can help you control your Carbs count. You can also use products such as almond flour as an alternative to regular flour.

Fruits

You can eat fruits on the keto diet but keep in moderation. Some fruits retract you from reaching ketosis. Berries though, are the most advantageous as they are packed with nutrition and hold a low level in sugar.

What to avoid

To reach ketosis successfully, do your best to prevent and rid your body of foods that will hold you back from your goal. Most foods to avoid are high in Carbsand do not allow your body to burn fat for energy. You should avoid these foods:

Root Vegetables

Vegetables that grow and get pulled from the ground are high in Carbsand take you away from ketosis. Such vegetables include potatoes, beets, radishes, carrots, onions, and parsnips.

Sweet Fruits

While following the ketogenic diet, you should avoid most fruits. Fruits contain fructose (similar to glucose) and are bad for reaching ketosis. Not only avoid fruits; stay away from products made with fresh fruit, such as juices and extracts. If you eat fruits, then keep it in moderation.

Grains

Obviously, avoid all foods made with processed grains. Grains contain additives that can negatively affect your insulin levels. Such grains include bread, pasta, cakes, breadcrumbs, cookies, and pastries.

Diet Soda

Diet soda claims not to contain sugars or carbs; it contains artificial sweeteners equally as detrimental as regular sugar. Artificial sweeteners enhance your Carbs intake and prevent you from reaching the metabolic state of ketosis.

Alcohol

Most alcohol beverages consist of none, or low carbs, but can still be bad for a keto lifestyle. Alcohol prevents the fat burning process or dramatically slows it down, because your body will need to process the alcohol first before the fat. To be successful with this diet, limit your alcohol intake.

Processed Foods

Avoid processed or packaged foods. Such foods are packed with artificial additives that can stray you from ketosis. Instead of choosing processed foods, pick organic and real ingredients. Opinions differ between some individuals and sources, but you get the concept. The ketogenic diet and instant pot have plenty of lot in common. It can be used together to make fast, tasty, and healthy dishes that will improve your life. Since the keto diet asks you to avoid greasy foods, the instant pot helps by softening up foods using pressure and heat. With that being said, let's use the instant pot to prepare ketogenic meals for better health.

Getting started tips

Gradually follow the ketogenic diet

A common mistake of many when starting the ketogenic diet is immediately eliminating Carbs. Doing this is not healthy for your body. While this may work in the short term, doing this can cause serious health problems over the long-term.

Give yourself time to maneuver into the keto lifestyle by making small but essential changes, like giving up one carb source every week or so. It's critical to give your body time to adjust to changes. An excellent way to overcome transition discomfort is to replace a healthy nutrient source to your diet for every unhealthy one. For example, if you use all-purpose flour, start substituting it with almond flour or coconut flour.

Drink plenty of water

When you start the ketogenic diet, your body will have a difficult time keeping the proper amount of water you need, so staying perfectly hydrated is the best way to go about it. Drink eight, 8-ounce glasses, which is equivalent to 2 liters every day. To know if you are well hydrated is to determine the color of your urine. Whenever your urine is light yellow or clear, you are properly hydrated. During a ketogenic diet, your body lose glycogen store and these glycogens hold some water release through urination. Drinking tea, coffee, smoothie and plenty of plain water may help you to stay hydrated.

Turn your favorite foods into ketogenic foods

Thinking of the foods you are not permitted to eat can become quite discouraging. Instead, learn keto-friendly versions of your favorite dishes. There are plenty of ketogenic cookbooks and internet recipes for tips and ideas on how to turn your favorite dishes into tasty ketogenic-friendly versions.

Following the ketogenic diet does not mean depriving yourself from your favorite meals, but about improving your diet and making it healthier. As the keto diet is high in fat, you will maintain all the flavors and texture from your favorite recipes. In many cases, the ketogenic diet has enhanced the flavor of many recipes.

Don't be afraid to ask for advice

If you have questions or confusions about the ketogenic diet, don't be afraid to ask for help. Ask professionals, ketogenic dieters, and maybe even certified nutritionists for advice, recipes, and experiences. You will be surprised by the experiences of others, and the information they share.

Be alert of alcohol consumption

You can still drink alcohol while on the keto diet without ruining the process. This is one of the great aspects of this diet. However, don't go overboard and drink all the time. It is preferred to go for unsweetened liquors, like scotch, tequila, vodka, whiskey, rum, and reduced-carb beer.

Be mindful of condiments and sauces

Not all condiments and sauces are healthy or ketogenic friendly. If you must use sauce and condiments, choose ones that are low in carbs, like soy sauce, lemon, salad dressings, mayonnaise, mustard, olive oil, and coconut oil (just to name a few).

In cases in which you can't tell if something is keto-friendly or not, you can always ask the server or chef. If they are not sure, it would be best to not use the sauce.

Be patient
Even though the ketogenic lifestyle is known for rapid weight loss, losing weight will take some time. Do not quit the diet when you are not experiencing quick results. Getting rid of fat will change throughout the day. Try not to get too worked up with a scale, instead be patient and trust that the ketogenic diet will help you lose weight.

Use vitamins and mineral salts
Foods high in Carbscontain many micronutrients, such as vitamins and minerals. When you stop eating Carbs, it can cause nutritional deficiency to your body. To help fight through this, you should use proper vitamins that can provide your body with nutrients.

Restock your fridge and pantry
If you are preparing to follow the ketogenic diet, the best way to begin is to rid the keto-unfriendly ingredients from your kitchen and restock with keto-friendly ones. This will make you more attentive and help you resist the urge to eat keto-unfriendly recipes.

Limit carb consumption
Keto diet is a low carb diet it recommends to consume below 25 grams of carbs daily. Eating low carb will keep your body in the state of ketosis.

Use MCT oils
Medium Chain Triglycerides (MCTs) are one of the healthy fats found in coconut oil. These healthy fats are quickly absorbed by your liver and convert it into ketones. It helps to maintain the level of ketosis in your body.

Sleep enough
While you are on keto diet enough sleep is very important. Sleep in a dark and cool room where temperature maintains at 65 F and sleep at least 7 hours daily at night.

Consume adequate amount of protein daily
Normally when you are on a keto diet your body burns fats for energy instead of a carb. In this process your body losses some muscles and fats. Maintaining your muscle mass, you just need to consume an adequate amount of protein daily.

Do exercise regularly
Regular exercise helps to maintain your blood sugar level and also reduce your weight. When you are doing exercise during keto diet your ketones level are increased.

Add extra salt to your diet
When you are on keto diet due to low carb consumption your blood insulin level decreases and it allows your kidney to release water and sodium from your body. Adding an extra 3 to 5 grams of sodium in your diet will also help to avoid electrolyte imbalance.

Clear out your kitchen of Carbs
Most of the people consume their favorite carb loaded food just because they fail to remove them from their kitchen. You must clean all Carbs from your kitchen pantry includes sodas, pasta, candy, bread, and rice.

Chapter 2: Breakfast

Breakfast Cheesy Sausage

This Cheesy Sausage is a low carb recipe that has nice the flavors! These pot pies are so delicious and are ideal for you.

Prep time: 20 minutes | Cooking time: 5 minutes | Servings: 1

Ingredients:
- 1 pork sausage link, cut open and casing discarded
- Sea salt and black pepper, to taste
- ½ teaspoon thyme
- ½ teaspoon sage
- ½ cup mozzarella cheese, shredded

Instructions:
1. Mix sausage meat with thyme, sage, mozzarella cheese, sea salt and black pepper.
2. Shape the mixture into 2 equal-sized patties and transfer to a hot pan.
3. Cook for about 5 minutes per side and dish out to serve.

Nutritional info per serving:
Calories 245 | Carbs 0.8 g | Fats 19.6 g | Protein 15.7 g

Tip: You can take this recipe with a hot drink.

Cauliflower Toast with Avocado

The combination of the cauliflower and avocado will definitely leave you wanting more. They have low calories and are high in flavors! Isn't that awesome?

Prep time: 20 minutes | Cooking time: 20 minutes | Servings: 3

Ingredients:
- 3 large eggs
- 3 big head cauliflower, grated
- 3 medium avocados, pitted and chopped
- 1 cup mozzarella cheese, shredded
- Salt and black pepper, to taste

Instructions:
1. Preheat the oven to 420°F and line a baking sheet with parchment.
2. Place the cauliflower in a microwave-safe bowl and microwave for about 7 minutes on high.
3. Spread on paper towels to drain after the cauliflower has completely cooled and press with a clean towel to remove excess moisture.
4. Put the cauliflower back in the bowl and stir in the mozzarella cheese and egg.
5. Season with salt and black pepper and stir until well combined.
6. Spoon the mixture onto the baking sheet in two rounded squares, as evenly as possible.
7. Bake for about 20 minutes until golden brown on the edges.
8. Mash the avocado with a pinch of salt and black pepper.
9. Spread the avocado onto the cauliflower toast and serve.

Nutritional info per serving:
Calories 127 | Carbs 9.1 g | Fats 7 g | Protein 9.3 g

Tip: Try different flavored fruits for more flavors.

Keto Avocado Toast

This recipe is so sweet that you might want to hide the left overs so that you can eat the following day! It is simply delicious!

Prep time: 5 minutes | Cooking time: 2 minutes | Servings: 2

Ingredients
- 1 tablespoon sunflower oil
- ½ cup parmesan cheese, shredded
- 1 medium avocado, sliced
- Sea salt, to taste
- 4 slices cauliflower bread

Instructions:
1. Heat oil in a pan and cook cauliflower bread slices for about 2 minutes per side.
2. Season avocado with sea salt and place on the cauliflower bread.
3. Top with parmesan cheese and microwave for about 2 minutes.

Nutritional info per serving:
Calories 141 | Carbs 4.5 g | Fats 10 g | Protein 10.6 g

Tip: Do not overheat because it will ruin your recipe.

Chocolate Chip Waffles

This recipe brings in the best things as concerns waffles; crunchy and crispy. Do not

wait any longer as you can prepare this recipe as soon as today!
Prep time: 30 minutes | Servings: 3
Ingredients:
- 3 scoop vanilla protein powder
- 3 pinch pink Himalayan sea salt
- 150 grams sugar-free chocolate chips
- 3 large eggs, separated
- 3 tablespoons butter, melted

Instructions:
1. Mix together egg yolks, vanilla protein powder and butter in a bowl.
2. Whisk together egg whites thoroughly in another bowl and transfer to the egg yolks mixture.
3. Add the sugar-free chocolate chips and a pinch of pink salt.
4. Transfer this mixture to the waffle maker and cook according to manufacturer's instructions.

Nutritional info per serving:
Calories 301 | Carbs 6.9 g | Fats 18.8 g | Protein 29.9 g
Tip: Strawberries are good for this recipe too, add them if you love them.

Egg Crepes with Avocados

This keto recipe is a very simple recipe to make! It is also rich in fresh flavors that make eaters want more of it!
Prep time: 15 minutes | Cooking time: 3 minutes | Servings: 4
Ingredients:
- 4 eggs
- 2 large avocados, thinly sliced
- 3 teaspoon olive oil
- 1½ cup alfalfa sprouts
- 4 slices turkey breast cold cuts, shredded

Instructions:
1. Heat olive oil over medium heat in a pan and crack in the eggs.
2. Spread the eggs lightly with the spatula and cook for about 3 minutes on both sides.
3. Dish out the egg crepe and top with turkey breast, alfalfa sprouts and avocado.
4. Roll up tightly and serve warm.

Nutritional info per serving:
Calories 372 | Carbs 9.3 g | Fats 25.9 g | Protein 27.2 g

Ham and Cheese Pockets

This is a great recipe to kick-start your day. It is creamy and s very nutritious.
Prep time: 30 minutes | Cooking time: 20 minutes | Servings: 3
Ingredients:
- 3 oz cream cheese
- 1 cup mozzarella cheese, shredded
- 3 tablespoons flax meal
- 4 oz provolone cheese slices
- 6 oz ham

Instructions:
1. Preheat the oven to 400°F and line a baking sheet with parchment paper.
2. Microwave mozzarella cheese and cream cheese for about 1 minute.
3. Stir in the flax meal and combine well to make the dough.
4. Roll the dough and add provolone cheese slices and ham.
5. Fold the dough like an envelope, seal it and poke some holes in it.
6. Place on the baking sheet and transfer to the oven.
7. Bake for about 20 minutes until golden brown and remove from the oven.
8. Allow it to cool and cut in half while still hot to serve.

Nutritional info per serving:
Calories 361 | Carbs 7.9 g | Fats 27.6 g | Protein 24.8 g
Tip: Timing is the key to getting a perfect end-product when making this recipe.

Clementine and Pistachio Ricotta

This is a quick breakfast recipe to make and it is also easy. You will love every bit of it.
Prep time: 10 minutes | Servings: 3
Ingredients:
- 3 teaspoons pistachios, chopped
- 1 cup ricotta
- 6 strawberries
- 2 tablespoon butter, melted
- 3 clementine, peeled and segmented

Instructions:
1. Divide the ricotta into 2 serving bowls.
2. Top with clementine segments, strawberries, pistachios and butter to serve.

Nutritional info per serving:

Calories 311 | Carbs 12.7 g | Fats 25.1 g | Protein 10.7 g
Tip: Try topping with different fruits or veggies to get different flavors.

Avo-Tacos

Keto Avo-Tacos a sweet and deliciously crunchy that you will enjoy them.
Prep time: 15 minutes | Cooking time: 5 minutes | Servings: 4

Ingredients
- 30 milliliters, Avocado Oil
- 60 g, Cauliflower Rice
- 58 g, Walnuts or Pecans, crushed
- 14 g, Chipotle Chili, chopped
- 14 g, Jalapeno Pepper, minced
- 20 g Onions, chopped
- 2.5 g Cumin
- 2.5 g salt, sea salt preferred
- 100 g, Tomato, ripe, diced
- 2 tablespoons, Lime Juice

Instructions:
1. Start by grabbing a bowl and putting the salsa ingredients together; in a small bowl, you'll need the diced tomatoes, jalapeno, the onion, and half of the lime. If you want, you can add in a bit of cilantro to give it a bit more freshness, and don't forget to add the salt!
2. Once you're done, put a frying pan on medium heat and add the avocado oil and let it heat.
3. In the meantime, you can get together the rest of the ingredients, including the cauliflower-rice (which you can totally make at home if you want--it's a 5-minute blend job), and toss in everything but the avocado, and cook on low to medium heat for about 5 minutes.
4. Add the mixture to the avocado halves and top with salsa and munch away!

Nutritional info per serving:
Calories 179 | Carbs 13 g | Fats 28.24 g | Protein 4 g
Tip: You can also use nuts of your choice in place of the listed ones.

The Asian Chickpea Pancake

This is so easy to make that you'll want to make it every week.
Prep time: 5 minutes | Cooking time: 10 minutes | Servings: 1

Ingredients:
- 34 grams Green Onion, chopped
- 34 grams Red Pepper, thinly sliced
- 70 grams Chickpea Powder
- 1.5 grams, Garlic Powder
- 1.25 grams, Baking Powder
- 1.5 grams, Salt
- 0.25 gram, Chili Flakes

Instructions
1. This chickpea pancake is super easy. Take your vegetables, prep them, then mix everything else, starting from the chickpea flour to the chili flakes in a bowl. Whisk until you see air bubbles, just like you would for a normal pancake.
2. Add the chopped veggies and after one final stir, add the mixture to a preheated skillet and allow it to spread evenly over the pan for about 5 minutes. Once the underside is cooked through, flip and let it cook for an additional 5 minutes, and once you are done, simply plate and serve.

Nutritional info per serving:
Calories 227 | Carbs 38 g | Fats 3.6 g | Protein 12 g
Tip: Try using different veggies for an amazing twist in flavor.

Overnight Oat Bowl

Oats are a favorite to many because they are so sweet and this recipe is no exception!
Prep time: 10 minutes | Cooking time: 10 minutes | Servings: 2

Ingredients
- 15 grams, Chia Seeds
- 75 grams, Hemp Hearts
- 14 grams, Sweetener
- ½ blueberries
- 2/3 Cup, Coconut Milk
- ¼ grams, Vanilla Extract/Vanilla Bean
- 1.25 grams of Salt

Instructions
1. Thoroughly mix in all of your ingredients and allow the bowl to sit overnight in a covered container to avoid evaporation. You want the oats to sit for at least 8 hours, so if you have a long night ahead of you, plan accordingly.

Nutritional info per serving:

Calories 634 | Carbs 17 g | Fats 52.32 g | Protein 27.75 g
Tip: Resting for 8 hours enriches this recipe with flavors.

Coconut Crepes

Coconut crepes, in addition to being super delicious, also happen to be very easy to whip up.
Prep time: 10 minutes | Cooking time: 8 minutes | Servings: 3

Ingredients
- 15 grams Virgin Coconut Oil
- ¼ cup, Almond Milk
- ¼ cup, Coconut Milk
- ¼ grams, Vanilla Essence
- 30 grams, Coconut Flour
- 15 grams, Almond Meal
- 1 cup Applesauce

Instructions
1. Dump all of your ingredients into one large bowl and whisk until smooth. Then set aside for ten minutes to allow the liquid to absorb into the flour. In the meantime, lightly oil a frying pan on the stove, and pour in the batter and spread until the pan is coated with a thin layer.
2. Cook until the crepe starts to get crispy, and flip. Another minute on the stove, and you are ready to serve alongside your toppings of choice or course.

Nutritional info per serving:
Calories 437 | Carbs 12.15 g | Fats 16.54 g | Protein 1 g
Tip: When you set aside for 10 minutes to allow the liquid to absorb into the flour, your crepes become more delicious.

Matcha Avocado Pancakes

This is a common recipe that is loved by many because its taste is amazing! You need to make this delicious recipe and you will love it all the way!
Prep time: 10 minutes | Cooking time: 5 minutes | Servings: 6

Ingredients:
- 1 cup Almond Flour
- 1 medium-sized avocado, mashed
- 1 cup Coconut Milk
- 1 tbsp Matcha Powder
- ½ tsp Baking Soda
- ¼ tsp Salt

Instructions:
1. Mix all ingredients into a batter.
2. To thin the mixture out, add water as need be.
3. Lightly oil a non-stick pan.
4. Scoop about a third cup of the batter and cook over medium heat until bubbly on the surface (about 2-3 minutes).
5. Cook for 1 minute on the other side.

Nutritional info per serving:
Calories 179 | Carbs 5 g | Fats 14 g | Protein 1 g
Tip: Cook over medium heat for the best results.

Low-Carb Breakfast "Couscous"

This recipe is very easy to prepare and also takes a very short time to get ready!
Prep time: 10 minutes | Cooking time: 2 minutes | Servings: 4

Ingredients:
- 200 grams Cauliflower, riced
- 30 g Strawberries
- 20 g Almonds
- 20 g Flax Seeds
- 60 g Mandarin Segments
- 1 cup Coconut Milk
- 1 tbsp. Erythritol
- ¼ tsp. Cinnamon Powder
- 3 tbsp. Rose Water

Instructions:
1. Mix all ingredients in a bowl (microwave safe).
2. Cook for 2 minutes at 30-second intervals.

Nutritional info per serving:
Calories 490 | Carbs 9 g | Fats 17 g | Protein 3 g
Tip: You can alternatively use an oven

Gingerbread-Spiced Breakfast Smoothie

This smoothie will spice up your morning and day and fill you with energy all day.
Prep time: 2 minutes | Cooking time: 0 minutes | Servings: 2

Ingredients:
- 1 cup Coconut Milk
- 1 bag Tea
- ¼ tsp Cinnamon Powder
- 1/8 tsp Nutmeg Powder

- 1/8 tsp Powdered Cloves
- 1/3 cup Chia Seeds
- 2 tbsp Flax Seeds

Instructions:
1. Place the teabag in a cup and pour in hot water. Allow to steep for a few minutes.
2. Pour the tea into a blender together with the rest of the ingredients. Process until smooth.

Nutritional info per serving:
Calories 649 | Carbs 10 g | Fats 46 g | Protein 6 g

Vegan Breakfast Muffins

Prep time: 5 minutes | Cooking time: 3 minutes | Servings: 3

Ingredients:
- 2 tbsp Almond Flour
- ½ tsp Baking Powder
- ½ tsp Salt
- 2 tbsp Ground Flax Seeds
- ¼ cup Coconut Milk
- 3 tbsp Avocado Oil

Instructions:
1. Whisk together almond flour, ground flax, baking powder, and salt in a bowl.
2. Stir in coconut milk
3. Heat avocado oil in a non-stick pan.
4. Ladle in the batter and cook for 2-3 minutes per side.

Nutritional info per serving:
Calories 194 | Carbs 2 g | Fats 21 g | Protein 1 g

Vegan Breakfast Biscuits

This recipe strikes a nutritional balance and also is so much enjoyable for everyone. It does not take long to get prepared

Prep time: 10 minutes | Cooking time: 10 minutes | Servings: 6

Ingredients:
- 1.5 cups Almond Flour
- 1 tbsp Baking Powder
- ¼ tsp Salt
- ½ tsp Onion Powder
- ½ cup Coconut Milk
- ¼ cup Nutritional Yeast
- 2 tbsp Ground Flax Seeds
- ¼ cup Olive Oil

Instructions:
1. Preheat oven to 450ºF.
2. Whisk together all ingredients in a bowl.
3. Divide the batter into a pre-greased muffin tin.
4. Bake for 10 minutes.

Nutritional info per serving:
Calories 406 | Carbs 10 g | Fats 28 g | Protein 7 g

Vegan Breakfast Sausages

This recipe could be the healthiest and the simplest that you will make ever! It takes just 20 minutes to get it ready and more so it is nutrients-packed!

Prep time: 15 minutes | Cooking time: 12 minutes | Servings: 4

Ingredients:
- 200 grams Portobella Mushrooms
- 150 grams Walnuts
- 1 tbsp Tomato Paste
- 75 grams Panko
- 1 tsp Paprika
- 1 tsp Dried Sage
- 1 tsp Salt
- ½ tsp Black Pepper

Instructions:
1. Blend all ingredients in a food processor.
2. Divide mixture into serving-sized portions and shape into sausages.
3. Bake for 12 minutes at 375ºF.
4. Serve.

Nutritional info per serving:
Calories 371 | Carbs 9 g | Fats 25 g | Protein 7 g

Quick Breakfast Yogurt

The Quick Breakfast Yogurt will make for a nutritious and enjoyable breakfast.

Prep time: 2 minutes | Cooking time: 8 minutes | Servings: 6

Ingredients:
- 4 cups Full-Fat Coconut Milk
- 2 tbsp Coconut Milk Powder
- 100 grams Strawberries, for serving

Instructions:
1. Whisk together coconut milk and milk powder in a microwave-safe bowl.
2. Heat on high for 8-9 minutes.
3. Top with fresh strawberries and choice of sweetener to serve.

Nutritional info per serving:
Calories 186 | Carbs 10 g | Fats 38 g | Protein 4 g
Tip: You can exercise your creativity here. Any flavor of ice or yogurt cream can be used for a base.

Spiced Tofu and Broccoli Scramble

The Spiced Tofu and Broccoli Scramble is just as easy as scrambled eggs and perfect for those who don't like eggs. Plus, the tofu takes on the flavors of the recipe.
Prep time: 5 minutes | Cooking time: 3 minutes | Servings: 3
Ingredients:
- 400 grams Firm Tofu, drained and pressed
- 1 tbsp Tamari
- 1 tbsp Garlic Powder
- 2 tsp Paprika Powder
- 2 tsp Turmeric Powder
- 150 grams Broccoli, rough-chopped
- 2 tbsp Olive Oil

Instructions:
1. Crumble the tofu in a bowl with the garlic powder, paprika, turmeric, and nutritional yeast.
2. Heat olive oil in a pan.
3. Sautee broccoli for a minute.
4. Stir in spiced tofu. Cook for 1-2 minutes.
5. Season with tamari.
6. Serve hot.

Nutritional info per serving:
Calories 331 | Carbs 7 g | Fats 17 g | Protein 16 g
Tip: You can add butter to make this recipe creamier.

Meat-Free Breakfast Chili

Many people do not believe that they can have chili for breakfast. This meat-free breakfast recipe is spicy and you love it.
Prep time: 10 minutes | Cooking time: 20 minutes | Servings: 4
Ingredients:
- 400 grams Textured-Vegetable Protein
- ¼ cup Red Kidney Beans
- ½ cup Canned Diced Tomatoes
- 1 Large Bell Pepper, diced
- 1 Large White Onion, diced
- 1 tsp Cumin Powder
- 1 tsp Chili Powder
- 1 tsp Paprika
- 1 tsp Garlic Powder
- ½ tsp Dried Oregano
- 2 cups Water

Instructions:
1. Combine all ingredients in a pot.
2. Simmer for 20 minutes.
3. Serve with your favorite bread or some slices of fresh avocado.

Nutritional info per serving:
Calories 174 | Carbs 9 g | Fats 9 g | Protein 18 g

Vegan Southwestern Breakfast

The Vegan South-western Breakfast consists of lots of healthy vegetables that will satisfy you and your family.
Prep time: 10 minutes | Cooking time: 5 minutes | Servings: 6
Ingredients:
- 1 small White Onion, diced
- 1 Bell Pepper, diced
- 150 grams Mushrooms, sliced
- 400 grams Firm Tofu, crumbled
- 1 tsp Turmeric Powder
- 1 tbsp Garlic Powder
- 2 tbsp Nutritional Yeast
- ¼ cup Chopped Green Onions
- 2 cups Fresh Spinach
- 1 cup Cherry Tomatoes
- 2 cups Baked Beans
- 2 tbsp Olive Oil

Instructions:
1. Sautee onions, bell peppers, and mushrooms until onions are translucent.
2. Add in the tofu.
3. Stir in the turmeric, garlic powder, and nutritional yeast.
4. Add green onions and spinach. Sautee for 1-2 minutes.
5. Serve with baked beans and cherry tomatoes.

Nutritional info per serving:
Calories 174 | Carbs 10 g | Fats 10 g | Protein 13 g
Tip: you can also add more vegetables that are fine enjoying.

Egg Roll Bowl

This keto recipe is one of the recipes that you are likely not to share with anyone! It is simply amazing!

Prep time: 5 minutes | Cooking time: 6 minutes | Servings: 2

Ingredients:
- 2 7-oz. packs shirataki noodles
- 1 tbsp. coconut oil
- 1 tbsp. sesame oil
- 1 tbsp. rice vinegar
- 1 12-oz. pack extra firm tofu, drained, cubed
- 1 red onion, diced
- 2 garlic cloves, minced
- 1-inch fresh ginger, finely minced
- 4 tbsp. low sodium soy sauce
- ½ cup red pickled cabbage, chopped
- ½ cup carrots, matchsticks or julienned

Instructions:
1. In a medium bowl, rinse the shirataki noodles with cold water, drain, and set aside.
2. Put a large skillet over medium-high heat.
3. Add the coconut oil and sesame oil to the skillet.
4. Add the rice vinegar, tofu cubes, and onions to the skillet. Stir-fry the ingredients until the onions start to caramelize.
5. Blend in the garlic, ginger, and soy sauce. Cook for a minute while occasionally stirring.
6. Add carrots and cook for 5 more minutes while stirring occasionally.
7. Take the skillet off the heat, divide the shirataki noodles over 2 medium bowls, top each portion with half of the tofu mixture and chopped cabbage, serve, and enjoy!

Nutritional info per serving:
Calories 319 | Carbs10 g | Fats 17.6 g | Protein 16.7 g

Tip: You can spice up this recipe by trying out a variety of vegetables.

Keto Breakfast Porridge

You can bet that it is awesome!

Prep time: 5 minutes | Cooking time: 5 minutes | Servings: 4

Ingredients:
- 1 cup Flaked Coconut
- ½ cup Hemp Seeds
- 1 tbsp Coconut Flour
- 1 cup Water
- ½ cup Coconut Cream
- 1 tbsp Ground Cinnamon
- 1 tbsp Erythritol

Instructions:
1. Combine all ingredients in a pot.
2. Simmer for 5 minutes, stirring continuously.

Nutritional info per serving:
Calories 402 | Carbs9 g | Fats 18 g | Protein 4 g

Keto Choco "Oats"

This keto recipe is among the fastest and easiest and this is the reason why you will love it! It is amazing and it tastes good with any diet!

Prep time: 5 minutes | Cooking time: 5 minutes | Servings: 2

Ingredients:
- 200 grams Cauliflower, riced
- 1 cup Coconut Milk
- 2 tbsp Flax Seeds
- 1 tbsp Erythritol
- 2 tbsp Cocoa Powder
- 1 tbsp Vanilla Extract
- 50 grams fresh Raspberries
- 1 tbsp Cacao Nibs

Instructions:
1. Combine cauliflower, coconut milk, flax seeds, erythritol, cocoa powder, and vanilla extract in a pot.
2. Simmer for 3-5 minutes.
3. Ladle into bowls and top with fresh raspberries and cacao nibs.

Nutritional info per serving:
Calories 564 | Carbs10 g | Fats 41 g | Protein 22 g

Tip: If you are not in hurry, you can simmer for longer time so that that it is rich in flavor.

Banana Hazelnut Waffles

Crisp and light, these Banana Hazelnut Waffles offer a sweet and crunchy option for your breakfast.

Prep time: 3 minutes | Cooking time: 5 minutes | Servings: 2

Ingredients:
- 2 tbsp Flaxseed Meal

- 1/2 cup Almond Flour
- 2 tbsp Erythritol
- 1 tsp Baking Powder
- 1 tsp Ground Cinnamon
- 2 tbsp Hazelnut Butter
- ½ cup Coconut Milk
- 1 tsp Banana Essence

Instructions:
1. Blend the ingredients until smooth.
2. Pour into waffle iron and cook for 3-5 minutes.

Nutritional info per serving:
Calories 316 | Carbs 9 g | Fats 31 g | Protein 3 g

Tip: For a different flavor, you can play with the different ingredients.

Vegan Breakfast Skillet

Who doesn't love this? I guess none. This vegan skillet offers you a nutritious and healthy meal that will make you start your day on a high.

Prep time: 3 minutes | Cooking time: 5 minutes | Servings: 4

Ingredients:
- 3 tbsp Olive Oil
- 400 g Firm Tofu, drained and crumbled
- 20 g Chickpeas
- 100 g Spinach
- 1 tbsp g Powder
- 1 tsp Paprika
- ½ tsp Turmeric Powder
- ¼ tsp Salt
- ¼ tsp Pepper

Instructions:
1. Heat olive oil in a skillet.
2. Add tofu and stir for about 3 minutes.
3. Stir in all the spices.
4. Add chickpeas and spinach. Saute for another minute.
5. Serve hot.

Nutritional info per serving:
Calories 271 | Carbs 10 g | Fats 19 g | Protein 18 g

Tip: You can top up with some veggies while serving.

Vegan Breakfast Hash

No matter the diet that you could be on, this meal tastes good. It can be made for anyone that is not on any diet and they will not be disappointed.

Prep time: 15 minutes | Cooking time: 5 minutes | Servings: 4

Ingredients:
- 1 cup Cooked Quinoa
- 1 cup Shredded Broccoli
- 2 tbsp Flax Seed
- ½ cup Coconut Flour
- 1 tsp Garlic Powder
- 1 tsp Onion Powder
- 2 tbsp Coconut Oil

Instructions:
1. Stir flax seeds with half a cup of water in a large mixing bowl. Leave for a few minutes.
2. Stir in all remaining ingredients.
3. Form the mixture into patties.
4. Heat vegetable oil in a pan.
5. Fry each side of the patties for 2-3 minutes.

Nutritional info per serving:
Calories 135 | Carbs 10 g | Fats 10 g | Protein 3 g

Tiramisu Chia Pudding

One thing that will make you love this recipe is the quickness with which you can whip it together! It so fast and it makes it good recipe when you do not have much time with you! It saves you time!

Prep time: 15 minutes | Cooking time: 5 minutes | Servings: 1

Ingredients:
- ¼ cup Chia Seeds
- 2 tsp Instant Coffee
- 2 tbsp Coconut Cream
- ¾ cup Water
- 1 tbsp Erythritol
- 1 tsp Powdered Cinnamon

Instructions:
1. Combine all ingredients in a mason jar.
2. Shake until well blended.
3. Chill for at least 20 minutes.

Nutritional info per serving:
Calories 112 | Carbs 9 g | Fats 9 g | Protein 3 g

Tofu and Spinach Frittata

The Tofu and Spinach Frittata is flavorful and filing. You can use your leftover vegetables to prepare this recipe.

Prep time: 15 minutes | Cooking time: 5 minutes | Servings: 4

Ingredients:
- 400 grams Firm Tofu
- 2 tbsp tamari
- 2 tbsp Nutritional Yeast
- 1 tsp Turmeric
- 1 tbsp Garlic Powder
- 2 cups Baby Spinach, chopped
- 1 Red Bell Pepper, chopped
- 2 tbsp Olive Oil

Instructions:
1. Combine tofu, tamari, nutritional yeast, turmeric, and garlic powder in a food processor. Blend until smooth.
2. Fold in the spinach and bell pepper into the mixture.
3. Brush an iron skillet with olive oil.
4. Pour the mixture into the skillet.
5. Bake for 25 minutes at 360F.

Nutritional info per serving:
Calories 236 | Carbs9 g | Fats 16 g | Protein 18 g

Tip: If you see like it's not ready after 25 minutes, add a few more minutes.

Fat-Bomb Frappuccino

This drink will brighten you up your morning!

Prep time: 15 minutes | Servings: 1

Ingredients:
- 2/3 cup Brewed Coffee
- ¼ cup Almond Milk
- 2 tbsp Erythritol
- 1 tsp Vanilla Extract
- 2 tbsp Coconut Oil
- ½ cup Ice Cubes

Instructions:
1. Blend coffee, coconut oil, vanilla extract, and erythritol until smooth.

Nutritional info per serving:
Calories 278 | Carbs6 g | Fats 28 g | Protein 1 g

Tip: Use the coffee when it is still hot.

Chapter 3: Soups & Salads

Instant Pot Beans & Ham Soup

This soup is filled with flavor and you will just not stop at one bowl.
Prep time: 15 minutes | Cooking time: 50 minutes | Servings: 6

Ingredients
- 1 cup Chopped onion
- 1 cup Dried black soybeans
- 1 cup Chopped celery
- 1 teaspoon Dried oregano
- 1 teaspoon Cajun seasoning
- ½ 1 teaspoon Salt
- Liquid smoke
- Hot sauce
- 4 minced garlic cloves
- 2 teaspoons all-purpose seasoning
- 2 smoked ham hocks
- 2 cups Water
- 2 cups Chopped ham

Instructions:
1. Add all of the fixings to your Instant Pot and choose the bean/chili function (30 min. high-pressure). Natural release for 10 minutes, and quick release the rest of the pressure.
2. Trash the bone and add the meat back in the soup. Roughly puree some of the soup with an immersion blender.
3. Enjoy piping hot with some hot sauce on the side.

Nutritional info per serving:
Calories 269 | Carbs13 g | Fats 14 g | Protein 21 g
Tip: If you do not like spices, you can remove them from this recipe.

Truffle Parmesan Salad

This paleo recipe is flavorful and so much fun when eating! It comes with spices and vegetables that make it super delicious!
Prep time: 15 minutes | Cooking time: 0 minutes | Servings: 4

Ingredients:
- 4 cups kale, chopped
- ½ cup truffle parmesan cheese
- 1 tsp. Dijon mustard
- 2 tbsp. olive oil
- 2 tbsp. lemon juice
- Salt and pepper to taste
- 2 tbsp. water

Instructions:
1. Rinse the kale with cold water, then drain the kale and put it into a large bowl.
2. In a medium-sized bowl, mix the rest ingredients into a dressing.
3. Pour the dressing over the kale and stir gently to cover the kale evenly.
4. Transfer the large bowl to the fridge and allow the salad to chill for up to one hour – doing so will guarantee a better flavor. Alternatively, the salad can be served right away. Enjoy!

Nutritional info per serving:
Calories 199 | Carbs10 g | Fats 16.6 g | Protein 3.5 g
Tip: Placing the bowl in a fridge is an important process for this recipe.

Cashew Siam Salad

It so fast and it makes it good recipe when you do not have much time with you! It saves you time!
Prep time: 12 minutes | Cooking time: 3 minutes | Servings: 4

Ingredients:
Salad:
- 4 cups baby spinach, rinsed, drained
- ½ cup pickled red cabbage

Dressing:
- 1-inch piece ginger, finely chopped
- 1 tsp. chili garlic paste
- 1 tbsp. soy sauce
- ½ tbsp. rice vinegar
- 1 tbsp. sesame oil
- 3 tbsp. avocado oil

Toppings:
- ½ cup raw cashews, unsalted
- ¼ cup fresh cilantro, chopped

Instructions:
1. Put the spinach and red cabbage in a large bowl. Toss to combine and set the salad aside.
2. Toast the cashews in a frying pan, occasionally stirring until the cashews are golden brown. This should take about 3 minutes. Turn off the heat and set the frying pan aside.

3. Mix all the dressing ingredients in a medium-sized bowl and use a spoon to mix them into a smooth dressing.
4. Pour the dressing on salad and top with the toasted cashews.
5. Toss the salad to combine all ingredients and transfer the large bowl to the fridge. Allow up to one hour to chill the salad– doing so will guarantee a better flavor. Alternatively, the salad can be served right away, topped with the optional cilantro. Enjoy!

Nutritional info per serving:
Calories 236 | Carbs 4 g | Fats 21.6 g | Protein 4.2 g
Tip: When making salad, you can try adding different ingredients for a rich flavor.

Kelp noodle salad

This keto recipe is flavorful and so much fun when eating! It comes with spices and vegetables that make it super delicious!
Prep time: 10 minutes | Cooking time: 0 minutes | Servings: 4

Salad Ingredients;
- 3 green onions (sliced)
- 1 (11oz/340g) pack kelp noodles
- 1 cucumber (julienned)
- ¼ cup carrots (grated)
- ½ cup cashews (crushed)
- 0.5 oz. cilantro (minced)

Dressing ingredients;
- 2.3oz almond butter
- 1 garlic clove (minced)
- 1 tablespoon tamari/ coconut aminos
- 1 tablespoon swerve
- 2 tablespoons lime juice
- 1 teaspoon chili oil/ chili infused extra-virgin olive oil
- 1 teaspoon ginger root (grated)
- 1 teaspoon sesame oil
- Red pepper flakes (pinch)
- Sea salt (pinch).

Ingredients:
1. In a bowl mix the salad ingredients.
2. In a jar, mix the dressing ingredients. (seal the jar and shake to mix well)
3. Pour the dressing into the initial bowl.
4. Toss to mix and serve.

Nutritional info per serving:
Calories 240 | Carbs 4.6 g | Fat 11 g | Protein 7 g
Tip: Shaking to mix is really important because it makes the recipe come out very good.

Tasty Green Salad

One thing that will make you love this recipe is the quickness with which you can whip it together!
Prep time: 6 minutes | Cooking time: 0 minutes | Servings: 3

Ingredients:
- 4 teaspoons white wine vinegar
- ½ cup cherry tomatoes, halved
- 2 teaspoons olive oil
- Dash pepper
- 1/8 teaspoon salt
- 2 teaspoons minced fresh basil
- 3 cups torn mixed salad greens
- ¾ teaspoon honey
- 1 tablespoon shredded Parmesan cheese

Preparation:
1. Whisk vinegar, fresh basil, olive oil, honey, salt and dash pepper in a small bowl until blended.
2. In a separate large bowl combine tomatoes and salad greens.
3. Drizzle with vinaigrette and sprinkle with cheese.
4. Enjoy your meal.

Nutritional info:
Calories:1092 | Carbs: 15 g | Fat: 86 g | Protein: 57 g
Tip: Try making different flavor by using lemon.

Asparagus and Artichoke Salad

It is so fast and it makes it good recipe when you do not have much time with you! It saves you time!
Prep time: 15 minutes | Cooking time: 45 minutes | Servings: 5

Ingredients:
- 20 tender, fresh green asparagus stalks (woody stem removed, rinsed)
- 8 fresh, medium artichokes
- 4 tablespoons extra virgin olive oil
- 2 cloves garlic, peeled and chopped
- 1 ounce chopped pistachio nuts

- 1 large egg white
- 4 teaspoons chopped green onions + 1 green onion for garnish, chopped
- Juice of 1 lemon
- Salt and white pepper to taste

Preparation:
1. Fill a large pot ¾ of the way with water; add half the lemon juice and a generous sprinkle of salt.
2. Trim the artichokes by removing the leaves until you get to the light-yellow leaves. Set the hearts aside.
3. Place the artichoke leaves in boiling water. Cook 45 minutes. Once boiled, rinse under cold water.
4. Place the artichoke leaves in a food processor. Add the remaining lemon juice, half a glass of water (4 ounces), a pinch of salt and pepper, pistachios, green onions, garlic, and egg white. Blend for 1 minute. Add the olive oil slowly. Continue to blend until smooth.
5. Cut up the artichoke hearts and arrange on a plate. Place the asparagus over the top. Drizzle the sauce over the artichokes and asparagus. Garnish with fresh green onions. Serve.

Nutritional info:
Calories 444 | Carbs: 10g | Fat: 1g | Protein: 13g
Tip: You can substitute asparagus with zucchini or Brussels sprouts.

Spicy Satay Tofu Salad

This recipe is loaded with lots of nutrition and flavor which is ideal for whole family or for any occasion!
Prep time: 8 minutes | Cooking time: 18 minutes | Servings: 2

Ingredients:
- 1 (12 oz. pack) extra-firm tofu, drained and cubed
- ¼ cup peanut butter
- ½ tbsp. smoked paprika
- 1 tbsp. sesame oil
- ¼ tbsp. red chili flakes
- 2 drops liquid smoke
- 2 tbsp. water
- 1 tbsp. black sesame seeds

Salad:
- 4 cups fresh baby spinach leaves, rinsed, drained
- ¼ cup fresh mint leaves, chopped
- 2 tbsp. lemon juice
- 2 tbsp. avocado oil
- ¼ cup roasted cashews, unsalted

Instructions:
1. Preheat oven to 395°F and use a parchment paper to line a baking tray.
2. Put the peanut butter, paprika, sesame oil, chili flakes, and liquid smoke into a large bowl.
3. Add the water to the bowl and mix thoroughly until all the ingredients are combined.
4. Put the tofu cubes in the bowl with the peanut butter mixture and stir gently until all cubes are evenly covered.
5. Transfer the covered tofu cubes onto the baking tray, spread them out evenly, and sprinkle the sesame seeds over them.
6. Bake the tofu cubes in the oven for about 20 minutes, or until browned and firm.
7. In a bowl, mix the salad ingredients together.
8. Take the tofu out of the oven and let the cubes cool for about 2 minutes.
9. Divide the salad and serve the tofu on top enjoy!

Nutritional info per serving:
Calories 656.1 | Carbs 5 g | Fats 54.4 g | Protein 29 g
Tip: You can replace roasted cashews with roasted peanuts.

Thai Chicken Coconut Soup

Tom Kha Gai is a staple in Thai restaurants, boasting sweet and sour flavors. The coconut really brings this dish to the traditional level, and adds the creaminess the soup needs.
Prep time: 15 minutes | Cooking time: 1 hour 15 minutes | Servings: 8

Ingredients
- 4 cups chicken stock
- 2 small cans full fat coconut milk
- 3 stalks lemongrass, bruised and cut into small pieces
- 1 nub galangal, peeled
- 3 shallots, sliced
- 3 cloves garlic, smashed
- 5 kaffir lime leaves

- ¼ cup three crabs fish sauce plus 1 tbsp.
- 1 tbsp. honey
- 3 tbsps. Lime juice
- 3 tbsps. Coconut oil
- 1 lb. cooked chicken, shredded
- 2 oz. carrots, sliced
- 2 oz. red bell pepper, sliced
- 4 oz. button mushrooms, sliced
- 2 tbsps. Scallion, sliced on a bias

Instructions:
1. Mix the stock and coconut milk in a large pot and heat on medium heat. Add the fish sauce and honey.
2. In a cheesecloth sachet, add the lemon grass, galangal (sliced thinly), shallots, garlic and kaffir lime leaves and drop it in the soup. Tie the sachet to the handle of the pot.
3. Bring the broth to a boil, then drop to a simmer and cook for 55-60 minutes, stirring occasionally. Remove the sachet when finished, pressing it against the side of the pot to release as much broth as possible.
4. Add the lime juice and oil, tasting and adding more juice or honey as needed.
5. Serve the soup by pouring it over the raw vegetables and shredded chicken in a bowl.

Nutritional info per serving:
Calories: 402 | Carbs: 10g | Protein: 12g | Fat: 36g
Tip: You can add parmesan cheese to make the soup creamy.

Ham And Green Bean Soup

One ham can give you enough meat of a lot of meals, weeks' worth even. This soup can be made from whatever leftovers you have, giving you another option with all of that leftover meat.
Prep time: 5 minutes | Cooking time: 20 minutes | Servings: 12
Ingredients:
- 2 quarts chicken stock
- 2 cups water
- 2 tbsps. bacon fat
- 2 cloves garlic, minced
- ½ yellow onion, chopped
- 1 lb. green beans, cut in half
- 1 lb. red potatoes, quartered
- 1 lb. ham, cubed
- 1/2 tsp garlic powder
- 1/2 tsp liquid smoke

Instructions:
1. Sweat the onions and garlic in a pot with the bacon fat until fragrant and translucent, 2-4 minutes. Add the water and stock to the pot and heat to a boil slowly. Skim whatever impurities float to the top.
2. Add the beans and cook 3-4 minutes until just tender, then add the potatoes, liquid smoke and garlic powder. Simmer until the potatoes are tender, 10-12 minutes.
3. Add the ham to the soup and heat through. Season as needed and serve.

Nutritional info per serving:
Calories: 158 | Carbs: 10g | Protein: 11g | Fat: 7g.
Tip: You can swap the chicken stock for vegetable stock.

Superfood Soup

We all know the benefits of eating the so called "superfoods" on a regular basis. This is a great way to get them in, and it's simpler than you might think.
Prep time: 5 minutes | Cooking time: 10 minutes | Servings: 6
Prep time: 20 minutes
Ingredients
- 1 head cauliflower
- 1 white onion, peeled
- 2 cloves garlic
- 1 bay leaf
- 1/4 lb. watercress
- 1/2 lb frozen spinach
- 1 quart chicken stock
- 1 cup coconut milk
- 1/4 coconut oil

Instructions:
1. Mince the onion and garlic and cook in a pot with the coconut oil until they are lightly browned. Add the cauliflower, cut into small pieces, then crumble the bay leaf into it and mix well.
2. Cook for 4-6 minutes, then add the greens and cook on high heat until just wilted. Add the chicken stock and bring to a boil. Drop to a simmer and cook until the cauliflower is just tender.
3. Add the coconut milk and season. Stir to combine, then turn the heat off and blend

with an immersion blender until smooth. Season and serve.
Nutritional info per serving:
Carbs: 6.8g | Protein: 4.9g | Fat: 37.6g | Calories: 392kcal.
Tip: Fresh spinach is also suitable for this recipe.

Avgolemono Soup

This Greek soup has chicken and lemon as its main flavor components. Normally, orzo pasta is included, but the keto staple of riced cauliflower makes a great substitute.
Prep time: 8 minutes | Cooking time: 20 minutes | Servings: 8
Ingredients
- 2 tbsp EVOO
- 1 yellow onion
- 4 cooked chicken breasts, skin off, shredded
- 6 cups chicken stock
- 2 cups water
- 1/2 cup heavy cream
- 2 lemons, juiced
- 1/2 head of cauliflower, riced
- 3 eggs
- 3 tsp dill, minced
- 1 tbsp. parsley, chopped

Instructions:
1. Cook the onions in a large pot with some of the EVOO. Season once they are translucent, then add the stock, water, cream chicken and cauliflower.
2. Add the minced dill and lemon juice, then taste and adjust the seasonings accordingly. Cook the soup for 8-10 minutes until the cauliflower is just tender.
3. In a small bowl whisk the 3 eggs, then temper them by adding a small ladle of the stock, slowly, to the whipped eggs, mixing constantly to bring the eggs to the temperature of the broth.
4. Remove the soup from the heat, then add the tempered eggs to the soup slowly, stirring constantly.
5. Let stand for 5-7 minutes, then serve with black pepper and parsley.

Nutritional info per serving:
Calories: 251 | Carbs: 4g | Protein: 20.7g | Fat: 16.3g

Tip: Ensure that you mix constantly. This ensure that the eggs won't become large chunks.

Barbecue Chicken Pizza Soup

Don't let the name fool you; this soup is loaded with flavor that actually works well as a soup, despite what you might think. Try it out for yourself and see!
Prep time: 8 minutes | Cooking time: 18 minutes | Servings: 8
Ingredients
- 1 whole chicken
- 1 red onion
- 4 cloves garlic
- 1 can stewed tomatoes
- 4 cups green beans
- 3/4 cup spicy barbecue sauce
- 1 1/2 cup shredded mozzarella cheese
- 1/4 cup ghee
- 3 quarts water
- Fresh basil, chopped

Instructions:
1. Cover the chicken with the water in a large pot, then season and simmer for 50-60 minutes, until the meat easily fall off of the bone. Make sure that all of the chicken is cooked. Reserve the cooking liquid, then shred the meat between two forks.
2. Small dice the onion then cook in a pot, in the ghee over medium heat with the minced garlic cloves. Once the garlic is fragrant, strain the stock into the pot and bring the mixture to a boil.
3. Clean and cut the green beans, then add them and the tomatoes to the pot. Season well and cook until the beans are just tender, 12-14 minutes.
4. Mix in the barbecue sauce and chicken, and season with salt and pepper. Garnish each plate with shredded mozzarella and fresh herbs.

Nutritional info per serving:
Calories: 449 | Carbs: 7.1g | Fat: 32.5g | Protein: 30.8g
Tip: The long period of simmering is important. So, don't use less time.

Spicy Cauliflower Soup

Spicy foods and cauliflower marry perfectly, not just in this soup either. Use the same flavor profile and roast the cauliflower instead and you have an awesome side dish!
Prep time: 5 minutes | Cooking time: 15 minutes | Servings: 6

Ingredients
- 1 head cauliflower
- 1 turnip
- 1 white onion
- 2 cups chicken stock
- 1 piece chorizo sausage
- 1/4 cup butter
- 2 tbsps. chives

Instructions:
1. Cut the cauliflower into small pieces
2. In a large pot, cook the onions in some of the butter until they just begin to brown. Add the cauliflower, season and cook for 3-5 minutes. Let the cauliflower carryover cook as the soup stands.
3. Crisp the diced chorizo in a separate pan, then add the turnip and cook, together with the sausage, 8-10 minutes.
4. Blend half of the soup with an immersion blender. When it is mostly smooth, season with salt and cayenne pepper.
5. Serve the soup with more chorizo, then serve with chives.

Nutritional info per serving:
Calories: 251 | Carbs: 7g | Fat: 19.1g | Protein: 10.7g
Tip: Creamy butter is an addition in order to make this recipe creamier.

Vegan Cream Of Broccoli Soup

Here's another example of a cream free creamy soup. The almond milk and cauliflower will help not only with texture, but with a nice, sweet flavor to counteract the vegetal broccoli.
Prep time: 5 minutes | Cooking time: 20 minutes | Servings: 4

Ingredients
- 1 tsp EVOO
- 1 yellow onion, sliced thin
- 1 head cauliflower
- 3 cups plain almond milk
- 3 cups broccoli, finely chopped
- 1 tbsp. onion powder

Instructions:

1. Cook the onions in the oil in a large saucepan. Season and cook until golden and soft. Add the cauliflower and almond milk, then cover and boil.
2. Drop the heat to a simmer and cook the mixture until the florets are soft, 8-10 minutes. Add half of the broccoli and warm through.
3. Pour the mixture for the soup into a blender, then puree until very smooth. Return the puree to the pot.
4. Add the onion powder and the rest of the broccoli. Season and cook, covered, on low heat for 10-12 minutes, until the soup is thick and creamy.
5. Serve warm.

Nutritional info per serving:
Carbs: 11.5g | Fat: 3.9g | Calories: 123 | Protein: 6.5g
Tip: You can add mashed avocado to this recipe to spice it up.

Cream Of Mushroom Soup

This is a classic soup that boasts a lot of savory flavor. Mushrooms are often a staple of a vegan diet, and in the keto diet they are a big player as well. This is a great way to use scraps if you're cutting a lot of mushrooms.
Prep time: 5 minutes | Cooking time: 27 minutes | Servings: 2

Ingredients
- 2 cups cauliflower florets
- 1 2/3 cup plain almond milk
- 1 tsp onion powder
- 1/2 tsp EVOO
- 1 1/2 cups button mushrooms, diced
- 1/2 yellow onion, chopped

Instructions:
1. Boil the cauliflower in a pot with the almond milk and onion powder. Season with salt and pepper, then drop to a simmer and cook until the cauliflower is just tender, 5-7 minutes. Blend this mixture until very smooth in a blender.
2. Sauté the mushrooms and onions in a separate pan in the oil. Cook on high heat, so that the vegetables can gain color and the mushrooms will leach out some of their liquid.
3. Add the cauliflower puree to the mushrooms after 7-8 minutes, then bring to a

boil. Lower the heat and cover, then cook until the soup is thick and creamy, 10-12 minutes. Season and serve.
Nutritional info per serving:
Calories: 95 | Fat: 4g | Carbs: 7.9g | Protein: 4.9g
Tip: Ensure that you do not overcook the cauliflower.

Cream Of Tomato Soup

Vegans are often found looking for a suitable substitute for cream in a variety of recipes. You won't even notice the cream is missing in this rich, flavorful soup. Roma and sun dried tomatoes punch up the flavor.
Prep time: 10 minutes | Cooking time: 0 minutes | Servings: 4
Ingredients
- 4 Roma tomatoes
- 1/2 cup sun dried tomatoes
- 1/2 cup macadamia nuts
- 1/4 cup fresh basil
- 1/2 tsp white pepper
- 1/4 tsp black pepper
- 1 clove garlic
- 1 quart hot water

Instructions:
1. Blend all the ingredients together until completely smooth. Use the heat generated by the blender's motor to gently warm the soup. Depending on the strength of your blender, this could be from 5-7 minutes. Season with salt and pepper.
2. Serve warm. It's that simple!

Nutritional info per serving:
Calories: 187 | Carbs: 7.7g | Protein: 3.5g | Fat: 15.9g
Tip: The left over can be stored for up to 3 days in a fridge.

Yellow-beet salad with anchovies

An awesome holiday treat, this low-carb friendly anchovies with yellow beets is truly a new flavor to try
Prep time: 10 minutes | Cooking time: 0 minutes | Servings: 2
Ingredients:
- 2 oz. anchovies
- Fresh chives
- ½ red onion
- 2 baby gem or endive lettuce
- 1 cup mayonnaise
- 8 oz. cooked yellow beets

Instructions:
1. Thinly chop the cooked yellow beets, onions and anchovies.
2. Mix in a bowl with mayonnaise.
3. Garnish using thinly chopped chives.
4. Serve in endive lettuce or baby gem.

Nutritional info per serving:
Calories: 326 | Carbs: 4.6g | Protein: 4.5g | Fat: 8.9g
Tip: You can add the red beets to this recipe.

Vegan Cream Of Broccoli Soup

Here's another example of a cream free creamy soup. The almond milk and cauliflower will help not only with texture, but with a nice, sweet flavor to counteract the vegetal broccoli.
Prep time: 6 minutes | Cooking time: 22 minutes | Servings: 4
Ingredients
- 1 tsp EVOO
- 1 yellow onion, sliced thin
- 1 head cauliflower
- 3 cups plain almond milk
- 3 cups broccoli, finely chopped
- 1 tbsp. onion powder

Instructions:
1. Cook the onions in the oil in a large saucepan. Season and cook until golden and soft. Add the cauliflower and almond milk, then cover and boil.
2. Drop the heat to a simmer and cook the mixture until the florets are soft, 8-10 minutes. Add half of the broccoli and warm through.
3. Pour the mixture for the soup into a blender, then puree until very smooth. Return the puree to the pot.
4. Add the onion powder and the rest of the broccoli. Season and cook, covered, on low heat for 10-12 minutes, until the soup is thick and creamy.
5. Serve warm.

Nutritional info per serving:
Calories: 123 | Carbs: 11.5g | Protein: 6.5g | Fat: 3.9g
Tip: If you are not a lover of broccoli, you can use Brussel sprouts

Cream Of Mushroom Soup

This is a classic soup that boasts a lot of savory flavor. Mushrooms are often a staple of a vegan diet, and in the keto diet they are a big player as well.
Prep time: 6 minutes | Cooking time: 30 minutes | Servings: 2

Ingredients
- 2 cups cauliflower florets
- 1 2/3 cup plain almond milk
- 1 tsp onion powder
- 1/2 tsp EVOO
- 1 1/2 cups button mushrooms, diced
- 1/2 yellow onion, chopped

Instructions:
1. Boil the cauliflower in a pot with the almond milk and onion powder. Season with salt and pepper, then drop to a simmer and cook until the cauliflower is just tender, 5-7 minutes. Blend this mixture until very smooth in a blender.
2. Sauté the mushrooms and onions in a separate pan in the oil. Cook on high heat, so that the vegetables can gain color and the mushrooms will leach out some of their liquid.
3. Add the cauliflower puree to the mushrooms after 7-8 minutes, then bring to a boil. Lower the heat and cover, then cook until the soup is thick and creamy, 10-12 minutes. Season and serve.

Nutritional info per serving:
Calories: 95 | Carbs: 7.9g | Protein: 4.9g | Fat: 4g
Tip: Use scraps if you're cutting a lot of mushrooms.

Spinach & Cauliflower Soup

This creamy spinach and cauliflower soup is packed with nutrients.
Prep time: 10 minutes| Cooking time: 10 minutes | Servings: 4 servings

Ingredients:
- 1 White onion (peeled, diced)
- 1 Cauliflower head (chopped)
- 2 Garlic cloves (peeled, diced)
- 1 Bay leaf (crumbled)
- 5.3 oz. Watercress
- 7.1 oz. Fresh spinach
- 4 cups Vegetable stock
- 1 cup Coconut milk
- ¼ cup Coconut oil
- 1 teaspoon Salt
- Ground black pepper – to taste

Instructions:
1. Place the onion and garlic in a soup pot greased with some ghee over medium flame and lightly brown it.
2. Add the cauliflower and bay leaf and cook for 5 minutes.
3. Mix in the watercress and spinach and stir cook for 3 minutes.
4. Pour in the stock and bring to boil, cooking until the cauliflower is tender-crisp.
5. Mix in the coconut milk, salt and pepper.
6. Remove from the flame and blend using an immersion blender.

Nutritional info per serving:
Calories 392 | Fat 37.6 g | Carbs 9.7 g. | Protein 4.9 g
Tip: Use kale in place of spinach

Oriental red cabbage salad

Make a superb side dish with a mixture of orange, fresh cinnamon, and dill combined with shredded red cabbage! This refreshing side is light and have attractive colors, suitable for holidays and other times.
Prep time: 5 minutes | Cooking time: 20 minutes | Servings: 4

Ingredients:
- ¼ tsp ground black pepper
- 4¼ oz. butter
- 2 tbsp. fresh dill, chopped
- 1 tbsp. red wine vinegar
- 30 oz. red cabbage
- 1 tsp salt
- 1 cinnamon stick
- 1 orange, juice and zest

Instructions:
1. In a mandolin slicer or a food processor, finely shred the cabbage.
2. Fry in butter on medium high for 10 - 15 minutes. Softly fry the cabbage until it becomes shiny and soft, but not too brown.
3. Add pepper and salt. Put in orange juice, vinegar, and cinnamon. Allow it to cook for 5 -10 minutes.
4. Finally, when serving or towards the end, top with zest and dill.

Nutritional info per serving:

Calories 310 | Fat 11.6 g | Carbs 10.7 g | Protein 5.9 g
Tip: Use any excess as a topping on a sandwich and enjoy!

Broccoli salad with fresh dill

Exceptional Broccoli all for you. This delightful natural super veggie is a flavorsome side dish. Broccoli combined with fresh dill is appetizingly tasty!
Prep time: 5 minutes | Cooking time: 0 minutes | Servings: 2
Ingredients:
- ¾ cup fresh dill
- 1 lb. broccoli
- Salt and ground black pepper to taste
- 1 cup mayonnaise

Instructions:
1. Mix all the ingredients together in a bowl.

Nutritional info per serving:
Calories 252 | Carbs 5.7 g. | Fat 10.6 g | Protein 10 g
Tip: You can make use of halved Brussels sprouts or cauliflower in place of the broccoli. Additionally, you can make use of frozen veggies, and all the nutrients are still intact even if the texture is a bit different!

Zucchini salad with eggs

Zucchini can be used as a replacement of potatoes in this spiced up and keto friendly makeover of the loved potato salad, giving you lots of creamy flavor without carbs!
Prep time: 10 minutes | Cooking time to: 15 minutes | Servings: 3
Ingredients:
- 4 hardboiled eggs, chopped
- 2 tbsp. butter or olive oil
- 3 tbsp. pickled jalapeños
- 1 cup mayonnaise
- salt and pepper
- ½ green bell pepper, the seeds removed
- ½ tbsp. Dijon mustard
- 3 oz. celery stalks, thinly sliced
- 1½ lbs. zucchini
- 2 oz. finely chopped scallions
- 2 tbsp. finely chopped fresh chives
- 3 oz. dill pickles

Instructions:

1. Into tiny pieces, about half an inch (1-1.5 cm) thick, peel then cut the zucchini. Remove the seeds with a spoon. Put in a colander, and then add salt. Let it sit for about five (5) to ten (10) minutes then with great care, press out the water.
2. In butter, over medium heat, for some minutes, Fry the cubes. Don't allow them to become brown, just a little bit soften. Keep separate to cool.
3. In a big bowl, combine the other ingredients and once it's cool, add the zucchini.
4. Finally, serve as a side dish, especially for barbecue.

Nutritional info per serving:
Calories 196 | Carbs 4.1 g. | Fat 2 g | Protein 11 g
Tip: If you don't like hardboiled eggs, then you can tryout another variation without eggs.

Low-carb fried kale and broccoli salad

You will certainly fall in love with this low carb broccoli salad. A mixture of garlic, creamy avocado, tasty fried kale, and spicy mustard gives you this heavenly delight!
Prep time: 5 minutes | Cooking time: 15 minutes | Servings: 2
Ingredients:
- 4 oz. kale
- 1 tbsp. whole-grain mustard
- 2 tbsp. olive oil
- 2 avocados
- ½ cup mayonnaise
- 2 scallions
- 4 eggs
- 1 pinch chili flakes
- 2 garlic cloves
- ½ lb. broccoli
- Salt or pepper to taste

Instructions:
1. Combine in a small bowl, mustard and mayo and then keep separate.
2. To your liking boil the eggs be it soft, medium or even hard-boiled. When they're done, transfer them to ice cold water Immediately, as this will make them easy for peeling. When they get cool, into two equal parts or quarters, have them divided.

3. Get the avocados divided, take out the pit and cut them up into pieces.
4. Finely slice the garlic. Heat the oil in a frying pan, and with care, fry the garlic slices. From the pan, remove the garlic and transfer to a paper towel for it to become crunchy. In the pan, save the oil.
5. Scrupulously chop the kale and broccoli. To the garlic-infused oil in the pan, add a scoop of butter. Now, for some minutes, on medium high heat, fry the vegetables until it becomes softened a little bit.
6. Finally, season with salt and pepper, and dish with eggs, avocado, and the mustard mayo. For extra taste and crunch, use fried garlic slices to complete the dish.

Nutritional info per serving:
Calories 201 | Carbs 5 g. | Fat 1 g | Protein 8 g
Tip: With baby kale or spinach, greens become very soft. To save you time when preparing, ensure you purchase them pre-washed.

Mixed cabbage coleslaw

This quick and easy side dish is light, fresh and colorful too. Enjoy it for picnics, block parties, and just at any time you wish!
Prep time: 10 minutes | Servings: 4
Ingredients:
- 1 cup mayonnaise
- ¼ tsp ground black pepper
- 4 oz. kale
- ½ tsp salt
- 8 oz. green cabbage
- 4 oz. red cabbage

Instructions:
1. Using a mandolin slicer, sharp knife, or a food processor, slice the cabbage into pieces.
2. Move into a bowl and then add the pepper, mayonnaise, and salt. Properly stir it and give it 10 (ten) minutes for it to settle.

Nutritional info per serving:
Calories 325 | Fat 27.6 g | Carbs 6.7 g. | Protein 9 g
Tip: The remaining can be kept refrigerated for about 3 (three) to 4 (four) days when you make a big batch.

Seafood salad with avocado

This tasty and fresh seafood salad is rich in protein, and it becomes a spicy low carb meal with the introduction of avocado, sour cream and mayonnaise.
Prep time: 20 minutes | Cooking time: 0 minutes | Servings: 2
Ingredients:
- 1 lb. cooked shrimp, chopped
- 1 tsp salt
- 2 tbsp. lime juice
- 1 lb. cooked salmon, bite-sized pieces
- ½ cup mayonnaise
- ½ cup avocados, chopped
- 1 garlic clove
- ¼ tsp white pepper
- 1/3 cup tomatoes, chopped (optional)
- ¼ cup red onions, finely minced
- 1/3 cup sour cream
- 1/3 cup cucumber, chopped

Instructions:
1. Combine in a mixing bowl, minced onion, mayonnaise, lime juice, sour cream, salt, garlic, and pepper. Keep separate.
2. In a bigger bowl, combine and mix together tomato, shrimp, salmon, cucumber, and avocado.
3. Over the seafood and vegetables, spray mayonnaise dressing and gently toss for it to mix together.
4. Before serving allow it to chill for twenty (20) to thirty (30) minutes.

Nutritional info per serving:
Calories 403 | Fat 12.6 g | Carbs 5.7 g. | Protein 9 g
Tip: You can add more green veggies if interested.

Jalapeno Bacon Cheddar Soup

This creamy and velvety soup is a delicious mixture of peppers, and bacon. And the cheesy goodness takes the texture of this soup to another level.
Prep time: 10 minutes | Cooking time: 30 minutes | Servings: 6
Ingredients
- 8 bacon slices
- 1 tablespoon olive oil
- 4 medium Jalapeno Peppers, stemmed and diced
- 24 fluid ounce chicken broth
- 4 tablespoons unsalted butter
- 1 teaspoon onion powder
- 1 teaspoon garlic powder

- ½ teaspoon ground cumin
- 1 teaspoon dried thyme
- ½ teaspoon celery seeds
- ¾ cup coconut milk, full-fat
- 8-ounce cheddar cheese, shredded
- 1 teaspoon salt
- ½ teaspoon ground black pepper

Instructions:
1. Cut bacon slices into 1-inch pieces.
2. Place a large pot over medium heat, add bacon pieces and cook for 3-5 minutes or until crispy, stir occasionally.
3. Then remove bacon pieces to a plate and reserve pot and bacon fat in it. Add jalapeno pepper to the pot and cook for 3-5 minutes or until sautéed. Then remove peppers from the pot.
4. Into a pot add broth, butter, onion powder, garlic powder, cumin, thyme, celery seeds and stir until mixed. Bring the soup to boil, then reduce heat to low and simmer for 15 minutes, stir occasionally.
5. Remove pot from heat and blend using an immersion blender or food processor until smooth.
6. Stir in cheese and coconut milk until well combined. Adjust seasoning and stir in jalapeno pepper and bacon pieces until just mixed.
7. Return pot to medium heat and simmer for 5 minutes or until heated through.
8. Ladle soup into serving bowl and serve immediately.

Nutritional Info per Serving:
Cal 552 | Fat 49.6 g | Carb 3.4 g | Protein 19.4 g

Tip: Always ensure the veggies do bot overheat.

Chicken Lime Soup

Mexican chicken lime soup is hearty, filling and extremely delicious. Make a large batch of this soup and store.
Prep time: 10 minutes | Cooking time: 45 minutes | Servings: 8

Ingredients:
- 6 chicken thighs, skinless and boneless
- 2 tablespoons olive oil
- 1 medium-sized white onion, peeled and chopped
- 6 teaspoons minced garlic
- 2 chipotle chiles, chopped
- 2 tablespoons adobo sauce
- 48 fluid ounce chicken broth
- ½ cup chopped cilantro
- 2 limes, juiced
- 1 ½ teaspoon salt
- ½ teaspoon ground black pepper
- 1 medium-sized avocado, peeled and pitted
- Crushed tortilla chips for serving

Instructions:
1. Rinse chicken pieces, pat dry and cut into 1-inch pieces, set aside until required.
2. Place a large pot over medium-low heat, add oil and let heat. Add onion and garlic and cook for 5-7 minutes or until onion is nicely golden brown.
3. Switch heat to high, push onion and garlic to the side of the pan and then add chicken to the pot. Cook for 5 minutes or until chicken is nicely golden brown, stir occasionally.
4. Add chipotle peppers, adobo sauce, and chicken broth and stir until just mixed. Switch heat to low and simmer soup for 15 minutes, skim off any foam.
5. After 15 minutes of cooking, adjust the seasoning and stir in cilantro and lime juice.
6. Ladle soup into serving bowls, top with avocado slices and tortilla chips and serve.

Nutritional info per serving:
Calories 317 | Fat 21 g | Carb 21 g | Protein 11 g

Tip: You can make your own broth at home and save on buying.

Jalapeno Pepper Soup

In this recipe, jalapeno pepper is presented with a new twist. It is amazingly comforting, creamy and cheesy.
Prep time: 10 minutes | Cooking time: 20 minutes | Servings: 4

Ingredients
- 4 large jalapeno peppers
- 4 bacon slices, rind removed and chopped
- 4-ounce cream cheese
- 4 fluid ounce coconut milk, full-fat

- 16 fluid ounce chicken broth
- 2 tablespoons tomato salsa
- ½ teaspoon garlic powder
- ¾ cup shredded cheddar cheese
- ¾ cup shredded jack cheese
- 2 teaspoons salt
- ¾ teaspoon ground black pepper

Instructions:
1. Remove stem from jalapeno peppers and grill on a griddle pan over medium-high heat until it begins to char and soften. Then peel the skin from the peppers and remove along with seeds. Chop flesh of pepper and set aside until required.
2. Place a medium saucepan over medium heat, add bacon pieces and cook for 5 minutes or until crispy. Remove cooked bacon to a plate and reserve pan.
3. Add chicken broth, cream cheese, and coconut milk and cook until cream cheese melts completely and the mixture is smooth, stir often.
4. Whisk in garlic, salsa, cheddar and jack cheese until incorporated. Add peppers, season with salt and black pepper and cook for 5 minutes until heated through.
5. Garnish soup with bacon and ladle soup into serving bowls.

Nutritional info per serving:
Calories 453 | Fat 37.76 g | Carbs 5.12 g. | Protein 17.74 g

Tip: You can alternatively use veggies to garnish

Chicken Chili Soup

Hearty chicken chili soup is a one pot meal. It is very simple and full of extraordinary flavors.

Prep time: 8 minutes | Cooking time: 4 hours | Servings: 6

Ingredients:

- 2 tablespoons butter, unsalted
- 1 large white onion, peeled and sliced
- 1 large green bell pepper, seeded and sliced
- 55-ounce chicken thighs, boneless
- 8 bacon slices, raw
- 1 tablespoon minced garlic
- 1 teaspoon salt
- 1 teaspoon ground black pepper
- 1 teaspoon dried thyme
- 1 tablespoon coconut flour
- 3 tablespoons lemon juice
- 8 fluid ounce chicken stock
- ¼ cup coconut milk, full-fat
- 3 tablespoons tomato paste
- 6 tablespoons sour cream

Instructions:
1. Plug in a 6 quarts slow cooker and place butter in the center of the pot. Then layer with onion and peppers and cover with chicken.
2. Cut bacon into bite size pieces and spread over chicken pieces and then season with salt, pepper, thyme and coconut flour.
3. Drizzle with lemon juice, chicken stock, coconut milk and tomato paste.
4. Cover slow cooker and cook on high heat setting for 6 hours until chicken is tender.
5. After 3 hours of cooking, uncover cooker and shred meat using forks.
6. Ladle soup into serving bowls, top with a heaping spoon of sour cream and serve immediately.

Nutritional info per serving:
Calories 317 | Fat 15 g | Carb 12 g. | Protein 32 g

Tip: You can add a few spicy ingredients to add the flavor to the soup.

Chapter 4: Vegetables & Side Dishes

Easy Cheesy Artichokes

Artichokes and shredded Monterey-Jack cheese combine very well in this recipe! Serve as a side dish or a complete vegetarian meal.

Prep time: 4 minutes | Cooking time: 10 minutes | Servings: 3

Ingredients
- 3 medium-sized artichokes, cleaned and trimmed
- 3 garlic cloves, smashed
- 3 tablespoons butter, melted
- Sea salt, to taste
- 1/2 teaspoon cayenne pepper
- 1 lemon, freshly squeezed
- 1 cup Monterey-Jack cheese, shredded
- 1/4 teaspoon ground black pepper, or more to taste

Instructions:
1. Start by adding 1 cup of water and a steamer basket to the Instant Pot. Place the artichokes in the steamer basket; add garlic and butter.
2. Secure the lid. Choose "Manual" mode and High pressure; cook for 8 minutes. Once cooking is complete, use a quick pressure release; carefully remove the lid.
3. Season your artichokes with salt, cayenne pepper, and black pepper. Now, drizzle them with lemon juice.
4. Top with cheese and serve immediately.

Nutritional info per serving:
Calories 173 | Carbs 9g | Fat 12.5g | Protein 8.1g

Tip: Top with fresh roughly chopped parsley.

Chinese Bok Choy

Bok choy, also sold as Chinese cabbage, is a nutritional powerhouse! In this recipe, it is flavored with butter, garlic, Five-spice powder, and soy sauce. Yummy!

Prep time: 4 minutes | Cooking time: 10 minutes | Servings: 4

Ingredients
- 2 tablespoons butter, melted
- 2 cloves garlic, minced
- 1 (1/2-inch) slice fresh ginger root, grated
- 1 ½ pounds Bok choy, trimmed
- 1 cup vegetable stock
- Celery salt and ground black pepper to taste
- 1 teaspoon Five-spice powder
- 2 tablespoons soy sauce

Directions
1. Press the "Sauté" button to heat up the Instant Pot. Now, warm the butter and sauté the garlic until tender and fragrant.
2. Now, add grated ginger and cook for a further 40 seconds.
3. Add Bok choy, stock, salt, black pepper, and Five-spice powder.
4. Secure the lid. Choose "Manual" mode and High pressure; cook for 6 minutes. Once cooking is complete, use a quick pressure release; carefully remove the lid.
5. Drizzle soy sauce over your Bok choy and serve immediately.

Nutritional info per serving:
Calories 83 | Carbs 5.7g | Fat 6.1g | Protein 3.2g

Tip: To make it spicier, add spicy ingredients.

Green Cabbage with Bacon

There are many recipes for a classic cabbage side dish out there. However, this Southern-style cabbage is one of the tastiest cabbage dishes you will ever try.

Prep time: 4 minutes | Cooking time: 10 minutes | Servings: 4

Ingredients
- 2 teaspoons olive oil
- 4 slices bacon, chopped
- 1 head green cabbage, cored and cut into wedges
- 1 cups vegetable stock
- Sea salt, to taste
- 1/2 teaspoon whole black peppercorns
- 1 teaspoon cayenne pepper
- 1 bay leaf

Directions
1. Press the "Sauté" button to heat up the Instant Pot. Then, heat olive oil and cook the bacon until it is nice and delicately browned.

2. Then, add the remaining ingredients; gently stir to combine.
3. Secure the lid. Choose "Manual" mode and High pressure; cook for 3 minutes. Once cooking is complete, use a quick pressure release; carefully remove the lid.
4. Serve warm and enjoy!

Nutritional info per serving:
Calories 166 | Carbs 7.1g | Fat 13g | Protein 6.8g
Tip: Add heavy cream to make this recipe creamy.

Warm Broccoli Salad Bowl

Prepare a crunchy, make-ahead broccoli salad that is sure to please the whole family! Broccoli is a great source of vitamins C, K, and E as well as dietary fiber and minerals.
Prep time: 10 minutes | Cooking time: - | Servings: 4

Ingredients
- 1 pound broccoli, broken into florets
- 2 tablespoons balsamic vinegar
- 2 garlic cloves, minced
- 1 teaspoon mustard seeds
- 1 teaspoon cumin seeds
- Salt and pepper, to taste
- 1 cup Cottage cheese, crumbled

Directions
1. Place 1 cup of water and a steamer basket in your Instant Pot.
2. Place the broccoli in the steamer basket.
3. Secure the lid. Choose "Manual" mode and High pressure; cook for 5 minutes. Once cooking is complete, use a quick pressure release; carefully remove the lid.
4. Then, toss your broccoli with the other ingredients. Serve and enjoy!

Nutritional info per serving:
Calories 95 | Carbs 8.1g | Fat 3.1g | Protein 9.9g
Tip: Do not exceed 5 minutes as this could spoil the deliciousness of this salad.

Creamed Spinach with Cheese

This dish is simply irresistible. Simply toss fresh spinach leaves with a cheese, spices and garlic to achieve your keto requirements.
Prep time: 4 minutes | Cooking time: 10 minutes | Servings: 4

Ingredients:
- 2 tablespoons butter, melted
- 1/2 cup scallions, chopped
- 2 cloves garlic, smashed
- 1 ½ pounds fresh spinach
- 1 cup vegetable broth, preferably homemade
- 1 cup cream cheese, cubed
- Seasoned salt and ground black pepper, to taste
- 1/2 teaspoon dried dill weed

Directions
1. Press the "Sauté" button to heat up the Instant Pot. Then, melt the butter; cook the scallions and garlic until tender and aromatic.
2. Add the remaining ingredients and stir to combine well.
3. Secure the lid. Choose "Manual" mode and High pressure; cook for 2 minutes. Once cooking is complete, use a quick pressure release; carefully remove the lid.
4. Ladle into individual bowls and serve warm.

Nutritional info per serving:
Calories 283 | Carbs 10.7g | Fat 23.9g | Protein 3.2g
Tip: Frozen spinach can also work if you do not get fresh ones.

Cheesy Spinach

The Cheesy Spinach is a favorite recipe for many families, loved by adults and children. Different people have different ways of making this recipe
Prep time: 15 minutes | Cooking Time: 15 minutes | Servings: 2

Ingredients:
- 1 tablespoon unsalted butter
- 1 small yellow onion, chopped
- ½ cup cream cheese, softened
- 1 (10-ounce) package frozen spinach, thawed and squeezed dry
- 2 tablespoons water
- Salt and ground black pepper, as required
- 1 teaspoon fresh lemon juice

Instructions:
1. In a skillet, melt the butter over medium heat and sauté the onion for about 6-8 minutes.

2. Add the cream cheese and cook for about 2 minutes till melted completely.
3. Stir in the spinach and water and cook for about 4-5 minutes.
4. Stir in the salt, black pepper and lemon juice and remove from the heat.
5. Serve immediately.

Nutritional info per serving:
Calories 301 | Fat 26.6 g | Carbs 10 g | Protein 8.9 g
Tip: Fresh spinach also work better.

Creamy Brussels Sprout

This keto friendly recipe is easy to prepare as it does not take lots of time to get ready. It is full of flavors because it used different ingredients.
Prep time: 15 minutes | Cooking Time: 15 minutes | Servings: 2

Ingredients:
- ¾ pound fresh Brussels sprouts, trimmed and halved
- 1 garlic clove, minced
- 1 tablespoon butter, melted
- 1 tablespoon Dijon mustard
- ¼ cup heavy whipping cream
- Salt and ground white pepper, as required

Instructions:
1. Preheat the oven to 450°F.
2. In a roasting pan, add the Brussels sprouts, garlic and butter and toss to coat well.
3. Roast for about 10-15 minutes, tossing occasionally.
4. Meanwhile, in a small pan, add the remaining ingredients over medium-low heat and bring to a gentle boil.
5. Cook for about 1-2 minutes, stirring continuously.
6. Serve Brussels sprouts with the topping of creamy sauce.

Nutritional info per serving:
Calories 125 | Fat 11.8 g | Carbs 3.6 g | Protein 1.6 g
Tip: You can never go wrong by following the instructions.

Broccoli Stir Fry

This recipe is made full of flavor and made from ingredients that are free of addictive. It also contains all the nutrients that are needed for various body functions. Try it today!
Prep time: 10 minutes | Cooking Time: 15 minutes | Servings: 2

Ingredients:
- 1 tablespoon coconut oil
- 2 cups broccoli florets
- 1 tablespoon low-sodium soy sauce
- ¼ teaspoon garlic powder
- Ground black pepper, as required

Instructions:
1. In a large pan, melt the coconut oil over medium heat and stir in the broccoli.
2. Cover the pan and cook for 10 minutes, stirring occasionally.
3. Stir in the soy sauce and spices and cook for about 5 minutes.
4. Serve hot.

Nutritional info per serving:
Calories 93 | Fat 7.1 g | Carbs 6.8 g | Protein 3.1 g
Tip: Heavy creamy can be added to made this recipe creamy.

Spicy Mushrooms

It has several but very amazing ingredients which make it deliciously spicy.
Prep time: 15 minutes | Cooking Time: 15 minutes | Servings: 2

Ingredients:
- 2 tablespoons butter
- ½ teaspoon cumin seeds, lightly crushed
- 1 small yellow onion, sliced thinly
- ½ pound white button mushrooms, chopped
- 1 jalapeño pepper, chopped
- ½ teaspoon garam masala powder
- 1/3 teaspoon ground coriander
- ½ teaspoon red chili powder
- 1/8 teaspoon ground turmeric
- Salt, as required
- 2 tablespoons fresh cilantro leaves, chopped

Instructions:
1. In a skillet, melt the butter in a skillet over medium heat and sauté the cumin seeds for about 1 minute.
2. Add the onion and sauté for about 4-5 minutes

3. Add the mushrooms and sauté for about 5-7 minutes.
4. Add the green chili, spices, and salt and sauté for about 1-2 minutes.
5. Stir in the cilantro and sauté for about 1 more minute.
6. Serve hot.

Nutritional info per serving:
Calories 147 | Fat 12.2 g | Carbs 8.1 g | Protein 4.4 g
Tips: You can substitute red chili powder with dry red chili if wanted.

Cauliflower Mash

Are you craving for something mashed and healthy? If yes, then this Do not forget recipe is what you exactly need. This recipe is packed with proteins, minerals and brimming antioxidants.
Prep time: 15 minutes | Cooking Time: 12 minutes | Servings: 2
Ingredients:
- ½ large head cauliflower, cut into florets
- 3 tablespoons heavy whipping cream
- ½ cup Parmesan cheese, shredded and divided
- ½ tablespoon butter
- Freshly ground black pepper, as required
- ½ tablespoon fresh parsley, chopped

Instructions:
1. In a large pan of the boiling water, add the cauliflower and cook, covered for about 10-12 minutes.
2. Remove from the heat and drain the cauliflower well.
3. Place the cauliflower, cream, ½ cup of cheese, butter and black pepper in a large food processor and pulse until smooth.
4. Transfer the cauliflower mash into a bowl.
5. Top with the remaining cheese, and parsley and serve.

Nutritional info per serving:
Calories 237 | Fat 16.9 g | Carbs 10 g | Protein 12.1 g
Tip: Reserve about ¼ cup of the cooking liquid for mashing.

Cauliflower Soufflé

Are you looking for a vegetable dinner that is relatively light and delicious? Look no further because this is what you need. This recipe is light and doesn't take long to prepare.
Prep time: 15 minutes | Cooking Time: 12 minutes | Servings: 6
Ingredients
- 2 eggs
- 1 head cauliflower
- ½ cup Asiago cheese
- ½ cup sour cream/yogurt
- 2 tbsp. cream
- 2 oz. cream cheese
- 1 cup mild/sharp cheddar cheese
- 1 teaspoon softened butter/ghee
- ¼ cup chives
- 6 slices crumbled cooked bacon – optional

Instructions:
1. Combine the two kinds of cheese, sour cream, cream cheese, cream, and eggs in a food processor. Pulse until smooth and frothy.
2. Chop the cauliflower, and add to the mixture (pulse 2 seconds at a time). Blend in the butter and chives. Empty into a 1 ¼ quart casserole dish.
3. Pour the water into the Instant Pot and add the dish. Secure the top and cook for 12 minutes using the high-pressure setting. Natural release for ten minutes, and quick release.
4. Garnish with the bacon.

Nutritional info per serving
Calories: 342 | Carbs 5 g | Fat 28 g | Protein 17 g
Tip: You can use any meat of choice to garnish.

Garbanzo and Spinach Beans

The Garbanzo and Spinach Beans are highly nutritious and delicious. They are sweet but not overly sweet.
Prep time: 5-10 minutes | Cooking time: 0 minutes | Serving: 4
Ingredients:
- 1 tablespoon olive oil
- ½ onion, diced
- 10 ounces spinach, chopped
- 12 ounces garbanzo beans
- ½ teaspoon cumin

Instructions:
1. Take a skillet and add olive oil, let it warm over medium-low heat.
2. Add onions, garbanzo and cook for 5 minutes.
3. Stir in spinach, cumin, garbanzo beans and season with sunflower seeds.
4. Use a spoon to smash gently.
5. Cook thoroughly until heated, enjoy!

Nutritional info per serving:
Calories: 90 | Fat: 4g | Carbs:11g | Protein:4g
Tip: Top with fresh veggies

Delicious Garlic Tomatoes

This is one of the recipes that are becoming so popular lately. There is usually one main reason as to why recipes become popular; the deliciousness!

Prep time: 10 minutes | Cooking time: 50 minutes | Serving: 4

Ingredients:
- 4 garlic cloves, crushed
- 1 pound mixed cherry tomatoes
- 3 thyme sprigs, chopped
- Pinch of sunflower seeds
- Black pepper as needed
- ¼ cup olive oil

Instructions:
1. Preheat your oven to 325°F.
2. Take a baking dish and add tomatoes, olive oil and thyme.
3. Season with sunflower seeds and pepper and mix.
4. Bake for 50 minutes.
5. Divide tomatoes and pan juices and serve.

Nutritional info per serving:
Calories: 100 | Fat: 0g | Carbs: 1g | Protein: 6g
Tip: Cooking less than 50 minutes will not yield a good outcome.

Mashed Celeriac

It contains minerals, vitamins, veggies and protein; a lot of nutrients way ahead than those received by most people in the world.

Prep time: 10 minutes | Cooking time: 20 minutes | Serving: 4

Ingredients:
- 2 celeriac, washed, peeled and diced
- 2 teaspoons extra-virgin olive oil
- 1 tablespoon honey
- ½ teaspoon ground nutmeg
- Sunflower seeds and pepper as needed

Instructions:
1. Pre-heat your oven to 400°F.
2. Line a baking sheet with aluminum foil and keep it on the side.
3. Take a large bowl and toss celeriac and olive oil.
4. Spread celeriac evenly on a baking sheet.
5. Roast for 20 minutes until tender.
6. Transfer to a large bowl.
7. Add honey and nutmeg.
8. Use a potato masher to mash the mixture until fluffy.
9. Season with sunflower seeds and pepper.
10. Serve and enjoy!

Nutritional info per serving:
Calories: 136 | Fat: 3g | Carbs: 11g | Protein 24g
Tip: you can alternatively roast the celeriac.

Apple Slices

Looking for something crunchy to cheer you up? Look no further. This is all you need.

Prep time: 10 minutes | Cooking time: 10 minutes | Serving: 4

Ingredients:
- 1 cup of coconut oil
- ¼ cup date paste
- 2 tablespoons ground cinnamon
- 4 apples, peeled and sliced, cored

Instructions:
1. Take a large sized skillet and place it over medium heat.
2. Add oil and allow the oil to heat up.
3. Stir in cinnamon and date paste into the oil.
4. Add cut up apples and cook for 5-8 minutes until crispy.
5. Serve and enjoy!

Nutritional info per serving:
Calories: 368 | Fat: 23g | Carbs: 9g | Protein: 1g
Tip: you can also bake the apple slices in the oven.

Cashew Sauce

This sauce is not complicated and is full of nutrients to keep you energized.

Prep time: 5 minutes | Cooking time: 0 | Serving: 4

Ingredients:
- 3 ounces cashew nuts
- ¼ cup water
- ½ cup olive oil
- 1 tablespoons lemon juice
- ½ teaspoon onion powder
- ½ teaspoon sunflower seeds
- 1 pinch cayenne pepper

Instructions:
1. Add nuts to your blender and process.
2. Add other ingredients (except oil and process until smooth.
3. Add a little bit of oil and puree.
4. Serve as needed!

Nutritional info per serving:
Calories: 361 | Carbs: 6g | Fat: 37g | Protein: 3g

Tip: Put in the fridge for about 30 minutes before serving.

Japanese Cabbage Dish

One thing that will make you love this recipe is the quickness with which you can whip it together!

Prep time: 25 minute | Cooking time: 0 | Serving: 6

Ingredients:
- 3 tablespoons sesame oil
- 3 tablespoons rice vinegar
- 1 garlic clove, minced
- 1 teaspoon fresh ginger root, grated
- 1 teaspoon sunflower seeds
- 1 teaspoon pepper
- ½ large head cabbage, cored and shredded
- 1 bunch green onions, thinly sliced
- 1 cup almond slivers
- ¼ cup toasted sesame seeds

Instructions:
1. Add all listed ingredients to a large bowl, making sure to add the wet ingredients first, followed by the dried ingredients.
2. Toss well to ensure that the cabbages are coated well.
3. Serve and enjoy!

Nutritional info per serving:
Calories: 126 | Fat: 10g | Carbs: 9g | Protein: 4g

Tip: Chill in the fridge before serving

Almond Buttery Green Cabbage

This good and sugar recipe is so fantastic and it's so satisfying because of its high fat content and needs just four ingredients to be prepared. Just when you need a treat, try it!

Prep time: 10 minutes | Cooking time: 15 minutes | Serving: 4

Ingredients:
- 1 ½ pounds shredded green cabbage
- 3 ounces almond butter
- Sunflower seeds and pepper to taste
- 1 dollop, whipped cream

Instructions:
1. Take a large skillet and place it over medium heat.
2. Add almond butter and melt.
3. Stir in cabbage and sauté for 15 minutes.
4. Season accordingly.
5. Serve with a dollop of cream.

Nutritional info per serving:
Calories: 199 | Fat: 17g | Carbs: 10g | Protein: 3g

Tip: Watch out on the cabbage as they could be ready in less than 15 minutes.

Brussels and Pistachios

This is a relatively easy recipe to make especially in huge batches and therefore it is ideal for potlucks or dinner parties.

Prep time: 15 minutes | Cooking time: 15 minutes | Serving: 4

Ingredients:
- 1 pound Brussels sprouts, tough bottom trimmed and halved lengthwise
- 1 tablespoon extra-virgin olive oil
- Sunflower seeds and pepper as needed
- ½ cup roasted pistachios, chopped
- Juice of ½ lemon

Instructions:
1. Pre-heat your oven to 400°F.
2. Line a baking sheet with aluminum foil and keep it on the side.
3. Take a large bowl and add Brussels sprouts with olive oil and coat well.
4. Season sea sunflower seeds, pepper, spread veggies evenly on sheet.
5. Bake for 15 minutes until lightly caramelized.

6. Remove from oven and transfer to a serving bowl.
7. Toss with pistachios and lemon juice.
8. Serve warm and enjoy!

Nutritional info per serving:
Calories: 126 | Fat: 7g | Carbs: 14g | Protein: 6g

Brussels's Fever

There is no better quick fix recipe than this.
Prep time: 10 minutes | Cooking time: 20 minutes | Serving: 4

Ingredients:
- 2 tablespoons olive oil
- 1 yellow onion, chopped
- 2 pounds Brussels sprouts, trimmed and halved
- 4 cups vegetable stock
- ¼ cup coconut cream

Instructions:
1. Take a pot and place it over medium heat.
2. Add oil and let it heat up.
3. Add onion and stir-cook for 3 minutes.
4. Add Brussels sprouts and stir, cook for 2 minutes.
5. Add stock and black pepper, stir and bring to a simmer.
6. Cook for 20 minutes more.
7. Use an immersion blender to make the soup creamy.
8. Add coconut cream and stir well.
9. Ladle into soup bowls and serve.

Nutritional info per serving:
Calories: 200 | Fat: 11g | Carbs: 6g | Protein: 11g

Garlic and Kale Platter

This recipe is spicy and very tasty. You will love it.
Prep time: 5 minutes | Cooking time: 10 minutes | Serving: 4

Ingredients:
- 1 bunch kale
- 2 tablespoons olive oil
- 4 garlic cloves, minced

Instructions:
1. Carefully tear the kale into bite sized portions, making sure to remove the stem.
2. Discard the stems.
3. Take a large sized pot and place it over medium heat.
4. Add olive oil and let the oil heat up.
5. Add garlic and stir for 2 minutes.
6. Add kale and cook for 5-10 minutes.
7. Serve!

Nutritional info per serving:
Calories: 121 | Carbs: 5g | Fat: 8g | Protein: 4g

Acorn Squash with Mango Chutney

Do you need to eat a squash? The Acorn Squash with Mango Chutney is a perfect solution.
Prep time: 10 minutes | Cooking time: 3 hours 10 minutes | Serving: 4

Ingredients:
- 1 large acorn squash
- ¼ cup mango chutney
- ¼ cup flaked coconut
- Salt and pepper as needed

Instructions:
1. Cut the squash into quarters and remove the seeds, discard the pulp.
2. Spray your cooker with olive oil.
3. Transfer the squash to the Slow Cooker and place lid.
4. Take a bowl and add coconut and chutney, mix well and divide the mixture into the center of the Squash.
5. Season well.
6. Place lid on top and cook on LOW for 2-3 hours.

Nutritional info per serving:
Calories: 226 | Carbs: 24g | Fat: 6g | Protein: 17g

Honey and Coconut Porridge

You can guess that this porridge is sweet. You can't hate it!
Prep time: 10 minutes | Cooking time: 8 hours | Serving: 8

Ingredients:
- 4 cups light coconut milk
- 3 cups apple juice
- 2 ¼ cups coconut flour
- 1 teaspoon ground cinnamon
- ¼ cup honey

Instructions:
1. In a Slow Cooker, add the coconut milk, apple juice, flour, cinnamon and honey.
2. Stir well.

3. Close lid and cook on LOW for 8 hours.
4. Open lid and stir.
5. Serve with an additional seasoning of fresh fruits.
Nutritional info per serving:
Calories: 372 | Carbs: 6g | Fat: 14g | Protein: 8g

Maple Glazed Carrots

The Maple Glazed Carrots are crunchily sweet.
Prep time: 10 minutes | Cooking time: 8 hours | Serving: 6
Ingredients:
- ¼ cup pure maple syrup
- ½ teaspoon ground ginger
- ¼ teaspoon ground nutmeg
- ½ teaspoon salt
- Juice of 1 orange
- 1 pound baby carrots

Instructions:
1. Take a small bowl and whisk in syrup, nutmeg, ginger, salt, orange juice.
2. Add carrots to your Slow Cooker and pour the maple syrup.
3. Toss to coat.
4. Close lid and cook on LOW for 8 hours.
5. Serve and enjoy!
Nutritional info per serving:
Calories: 76 | Carbs: 4g | Fat: 1g | Protein: 76g

Ginger and Orange "Beets"

This is an ideal recipe to cheer your lazy self!
Prep time: 20 minutes | Cooking time: 8 hours | Serving: 6
Ingredients:
- 2 pounds beets, peeled and cut into wedges
- Juice of 2 oranges
- Zest of 1 orange
- 1 teaspoon fresh ginger, grated
- 1 tablespoon honey
- 1 tablespoon apple cider vinegar
- 1/8 teaspoon fresh ground black pepper
- Sea salt

Instructions:
1. Add beets, zest, orange juice, ginger, honey, pepper, salt and vinegar to your Slow Cooker.
2. Stir well.
3. Close lid and cook on LOW for 8 hours.
4. Serve and enjoy!
Nutritional info per serving:
Calories: 108 | Carbs: 5g | Fat: 1g | Protein: 3g

Baby Potatoes

Potatoes are very nutritious and delicious and this recipe is no different.
Prep time: 10 minutes | Cooking time: 35 minutes | Serving: 4
Ingredients:
- 2 pounds new yellow potatoes, scrubbed and cut into wedges
- 2 tablespoons extra virgin olive oil
- 2 teaspoons fresh rosemary, chopped
- 1 teaspoon garlic powder
- ½ teaspoon freshly ground black pepper and sunflower seeds

Instructions:
1. Pre-heat your oven to 400°F.
2. Line a baking sheet with aluminum foil and set it aside.
3. Take a large bowl and add potatoes, olive oil, garlic, rosemary, sea sunflower seeds and pepper.
4. Spread potatoes in a single layer on a baking sheet and bake for 35 minutes.
5. Serve and enjoy!
Nutritional info per serving:
Calories: 225 | Carbs: 7g | Fat: 7g | Protein: 5g

Cauliflower Cakes

These are not the kind of cakes most people are used to. If you try them, you will not stop making them.
Prep time: 10 minutes | Cooking time: 10 minutes | Serving: 4
Ingredients:
- 4 cups cauliflowers, cut into florets
- 1 cup kite ricotta/cashew cheese, grated
- 2 eggs, lightly beaten
- 1 teaspoon paprika
- 1 teaspoon chili powder
- Sunflower seeds and pepper to taste
- ½ cup fresh parsley, chopped
- 1 tablespoon olive oil

Instructions:

1. Add cauliflower, cheese, paprika, eggs, chili, sunflower seeds, pepper and parsley into a large sized bowl.
2. Mix well.
3. Drizzle olive oil into frying pan and place over medium-high heat.
4. Shape cauliflower mixture into 12 even patties.
5. Once oil is hot, fry cakes until both sides are golden brown.
6. Serve hot and enjoy!

Nutritional info per serving:
Calories: 180 | Carbs: 6g | Fat: 8g | Protein: 8g

Coconut and Cauliflower Rice with Chili

Coconut and Cauliflower Rice with Chili is very delicious and god for any occasion.
Prep time: 20 minutes | Cooking time: 20 minutes | Serving: 4

Ingredients:
- 3 cups cauliflower, riced
- 2/3 cups full-fat coconut almond milk
- 1-2 teaspoons sriracha paste
- ¼- ½ teaspoon onion powder
- Sunflower seeds as needed
- Fresh basil for garnish

Instructions:
1. Take a pan and place it over medium low heat.
2. Add all of the ingredients and stir them until fully combined.
3. Cook for about 5-10 minutes, making sure that the lid is on.
4. Remove the lid and keep cooking until any excess liquid is absorbed.
5. Once the rice is soft and creamy, enjoy!

Nutritional info per serving:
Calories: 95 | Carbs: 4g | Fat: 7g | Protein: 1g

Fried Apple

The fried apple pieces are very crunchy.
Prep time: 10 minutes | Cooking time: 10 minutes | Serving: 4

Ingredients:
- 1 cup of coconut oil
- ¼ cup date paste
- 2 tablespoons ground cinnamon
- 4 apples, peeled and sliced, cored

Instructions:
1. Place a large sized skillet over medium heat.
2. Add oil and allow it to heat. Add date paste and cinnamon and stir.
3. Add the apples and fry until crispy, for 5-8 minutes.
4. Serve and enjoy!

Nutritional info per serving:
Calories: 368 | Carbs: 4g | Fat: 23g | Protein: 1g

Spaghetti Squash

This an easy recipe to make and it's worth the waiting time.
Prep time: 5 minutes | Cooking Time: 7-8 hours | Serving: 6

Ingredients:
- 1 spaghetti squash
- 2 cups water

Instructions:
1. Wash squash carefully with water and rinse it well.
2. Puncture 5-6 holes in the squash using a fork.
3. Place squash in Slow Cooker.
4. Place lid and cook on LOW for 7-8 hours.
5. Remove squash to cutting board and let it cool.
6. Cut squash in half and discard seeds.
7. Use two forks and scrape out squash strands and transfer to bowl.
8. Serve and enjoy!

Nutritional info per serving:
Calories: 52 | Carbs: 2g | Fat: 0g | Protein: 1g

Garlic and Mushroom Crunch

Just like the name suggests, this recipe is crunchy!
Prep time: 10 minutes | Cooking Time: 8 hours | Serving: 6

Ingredients:
- ¼ cup vegetable stock
- 2 tablespoons extra virgin olive oil
- 1 tablespoon Dijon mustard
- 1 teaspoon dried thyme
- 1 teaspoon sea salt
- ½ teaspoon dried rosemary
- ¼ teaspoon fresh ground black pepper

- 2 pounds cremini mushrooms, cleaned
- 6 garlic cloves, minced
- ¼ cup fresh parsley, chopped

Instructions:
1. Take a small bowl and whisk in vegetable stock, mustard, olive oil, salt, thyme, pepper and rosemary.
2. Add mushrooms, garlic and stock mix to your Slow Cooker.
3. Close lid and cook on LOW for 8 hours.
4. Open lid and stir in parsley.
5. Serve and enjoy!

Nutritional info per serving:
Calories: 92 | Carbs: 8g | Fat: 5g | Protein: 4g

Pepper Jack Cauliflower

This recipe is easy to make and is very delicious!
Prep time: 10 minutes | Cooking Time: 3 hours 35 minutes | Serving: 6

Ingredients:
- 1 head cauliflower
- ¼ cup whipping cream
- 4 ounces cream cheese
- ½ teaspoon pepper
- 1 teaspoon salt
- 2 tablespoons butter
- 4 ounces pepper jack cheese

Instructions:
1. Grease slow cooker and add listed ingredients.
2. Stir and place lid, cook on LOW for 3 hours.
3. Remove lid and add cheese, stir.
4. Place lid and cook for 1 hour more.

Nutritional info per serving:
Calories: 272 | Carbs: 5g | Fat: 21g | Protein: 10g

The Brussels Platter

This platter is the right meal for a light dinner. It will leave you happily satisfied.
Prep time: 15 minutes | Cooking Time: 4 hours | Serving: 4

Ingredients:
- 1 pound Brussels sprouts, bottoms trimmed and cut
- 1 tablespoon olive oil
- 1 ½ tablespoons Dijon mustard
- Salt and pepper to taste
- ½ teaspoon dried tarragon

Instructions:
1. Add Brussels sprouts, mustard, water, salt and pepper to your Slow Cooker
2. Add dried tarragon.
3. Stir well and cover.
4. Cook on LOW for 5 hours, making sure to keep cooking until the Brussels sprouts are tender.
5. Stir well and arrange.
6. Add Dijon over the Brussels sprouts.

Nutritional info per serving:
Calories: 83 | Carbs: 11g | Fat: 4g | Protein: 4g

Southern Salad

Southern salad is crunchy and very tasty. This salad brings a simple treat to your family dining table.
Prep time: 10 minutes | Cooking time: nil | Serving: 2

Ingredients:
- 5 cups Romaine lettuce
- ½ cup sprouted black beans
- 1 cup cherry tomatoes, halved
- 1 avocado, diced
- ¼ cup almonds, chopped
- ½ cup of fresh cilantro
- ½ cup of Salsa Fresca

Instructions:
1. Take a large sized bowl and add lettuce, tomatoes, beans, almonds, cilantro, avocado, Salsa Fresco
2. Toss everything well and mix them
3. Divide the salad into serving bowls and serve!

Nutritional info per serving:
Calories: 211 | Carbs: 6g | Fat: 16g | Protein: 10g

Kale and Carrot with Tahini Dressing

This is a quick fix dressing that you can as well enjoy it alone. It is just ready in 10 minutes only! Isn't that great?
Prep time: 15 minutes | Cooking time: 0 minutes | Serving: 1

Ingredients:
- Handful of kale
- 1 tablespoon tahnini
- ½ head lettuce
- Pinch of garlic powder

- 1 tablespoon olive oil
- Juice of ½ lime
- 1 carrot, grated

Instructions:
1. Add kale and roughly chopped lettuce to a bowl.
2. Add grated carrots to the greens and mix.
3. Take a small bowl and add the remaining ingredients, mix well.
4. Pour dressing on top of greens and toss.

Nutritional info per serving:
Calories: 249 | Carbs: 3g | Fat: 11g | Protein: 10g

Crispy Kale

This recipe is crispy and will excite you because of its nice taste.
Prep time: 10 minutes | Cooking time: 25 minutes | Serving: 4

Ingredients:
- 3 cups kale, stemmed and thoroughly washed, torn in 2-inch pieces
- 1 tablespoon extra-virgin olive oil
- ½ teaspoon chili powder
- ¼ teaspoon sea salt

Instructions:
1. Prepare your oven by pre-heating to 300°F.
2. Line 2 baking sheets with parchment paper and keep them on the side.
3. Dry kale and transfer to a large bowl.
4. Add olive oil and toss, making sure to cover the leaves well.
5. Season kale with salt, chili powder and toss.
6. Divide kale between baking sheets and spread into single layer.
7. Bake for 25 minutes until crispy.
8. Let them cool for 5 minutes, serve.

Nutritional info per serving:
Calories: 56 | Carbs: 5g | Fat: 4g | Protein: 2g

Summertime Veggies

This recipe gives an abundance of fresh vegetables like zucchinis, onions, tomatoes, fresh thyme, fresh basil red onions and many more. They are cooked slowly to perfection. You will enjoy this great recipe.
Prep time: 10 minutes | Cooking Time: 3 hours 5 minutes | Serving: 6

Ingredients:
- 1 cup grape tomatoes
- 2 cups okra
- 1 cup mushrooms
- 2 cups yellow bell peppers
- 1 ½ cup red onions
- 2 ½ cups zucchini
- ½ cup olive oil
- ½ cup balsamic vinegar
- 1 tablespoon fresh thyme, chopped
- 2 tablespoons fresh basil, chopped

Instructions:
1. Slice and chop okra, onions, tomatoes, zucchini, mushrooms.
2. Add veggies to a large container and mix.
3. Take another dish and add oil and vinegar, mix in thyme and basil.
4. Toss the veggies into the Slow Cooker and pour marinade.
5. Stir well.
6. Close lid and cook on 3 hours on HIGH, making sure to stir after every hour.

Nutritional info per serving:
Calories: 233 | Carbs: 14g | Fat: 18g | Protein: 3g

Caramelized Onion

These onions are cooked slowly on low until they turn golden brown and are very sweet. They can be very addicting once you start having them!
Prep time: 10 minutes | Cooking Time: 9-10 hours | Serving: 4

Ingredients:
- 6 onions, sliced
- 2 tablespoons oil
- ½ teaspoon salt

Instructions:
1. Add onions, oil and salt to your Slow Cooker.
2. Close lid and cook on LOW for 8 hours.
3. Open lid and keep simmering for 1-2 hours until any excess water has evaporated.
4. Serve and enjoy!

Nutritional info per serving:
Calories: 126 | Carbs: 15g | Fat: 15g | Protein: 2g

Kidney Beans and Cilantro

This recipe is tasty and also vegan friendly. It is a Mediterranean recipe that is very popular and I think you will not fail to love it.
Prep time: 5 minutes | Cooking time: nil | Serving: 6

Ingredients:
- 1 can (15 ounces kidney beans, drained and rinsed
- ½ English cucumber, chopped
- 1 medium heirloom tomato, chopped
- 1 bunch fresh cilantro, stems removed and chopped
- 1 red onion, chopped
- Juice of 1 large lime
- 3 tablespoons Dijon mustard
- ½ teaspoon fresh garlic paste
- 1 teaspoon Sumac
- Salt and pepper as needed

Instructions:
1. Take a medium-sized bowl and add kidney beans, chopped up veggies and cilantro.
2. Take a small bowl and make the vinaigrette by adding lime juice, oil, fresh garlic, pepper, mustard and Sumac.
3. Pour the vinaigrette over the salad and give it a gentle stir.
4. Add some salt and pepper.
5. Cover and allow to chill for half an hour before serving!

Nutritional info per serving:
Calories: 74 | Carbs: 16g | Fat: 0.7g | Protein: 21g

Broccoli Crunchies

This recipe, just like its name suggests, is crunchy and a little creamy.
Prep time: 10 minutes | Cooking Time: 3 hours | Serving: 4

Ingredients:
- 2 cups broccoli florets
- 2 ounces cream of celery soup
- 2 tablespoons cheddar cheese, shredded
- 1 small yellow onion, chopped
- ¼ teaspoon Worcestershire sauce
- Salt and pepper as needed
- ½ tablespoon butter

Instructions:
1. Add broccoli, cream, cheese, onion, cheddar to Slow Cooker.
2. Stir and season with salt and pepper.
3. Place lid and cook on LOW for 3 hours.
4. Serve and enjoy!

Nutritional info per serving:
Calories: 162 | Carbs: 11g | Fat: 11g | Protein: 5g

Buffalo Cashews

These buffalo cashews are not only spicy and crunchy but also packed with proteins. All your cravings will be satiated by these cashews.
Prep time: 10 minutes | Cooking time: 55 minutes | Serving: 4

Ingredients:
- 2 cups raw cashews
- ¾ cup red hot sauce
- 1/3 cup avocado oil
- ½ teaspoon garlic powder
- ¼ teaspoon turmeric

Instructions:
1. Take a bowl, mix the wet ingredients in a bowl and stir in seasoning.
2. Add cashews to the bowl and mix.
3. Soak cashews in hot sauce mix for 2-4 hours.
4. Pre-heat your oven to 325°F.
5. Spread cashews onto baking sheet.
6. Bake for 35-55 minutes, turning after every 10-15 minutes.
7. Let them cool and serve!

Nutritional info per serving:
Calories: 268 | Carbs: 10g | Fat: 16g | Protein: 14g

A Green Bean Mixture

The green bean mixture is a recipe that can be made for your family and it is very satisfying.
Prep time: 10 minutes | Cooking Time: 2 hours | Serving: 2

Ingredients:
- 4 cups green beans, trimmed
- 2 tablespoons butter, melted
- 1 tablespoon date paste
- Salt and pepper as needed
- ¼ teaspoon coconut aminos

Instructions:

1. Add green beans, date paste, pepper, salt, coconut aminos to the Slow Cooker, gently stir.
2. Toss and place lid.
3. Cook on LOW for 2 hours.
4. Serve and enjoy!

Nutritional info per serving:
Calories: 236 | Carbs: 10g | Fat: 6g | Protein: 6g

Cauliflower and Mushroom Risotto

The Cauliflower and Mushroom Risotto is creamy and rich in flavor and delicious.
Prep time: 10 minutes | Cooking time: 20 minutes | Serving: 4

Ingredients:
- 1 cup vegetable stock
- head cauliflower, grated
- 9 ounces mushroom, chopped
- tablespoons almond butter
- Sunflower seeds and black pepper, to taste
- 1 cup coconut cream

Instructions:
1. Take a saucepan and pour stock into it.
2. Bring it to boil and set it aside.
3. Then take a skillet and melt almond butter over medium heat.
4. Add mushroom to sauté until it turns golden brown.
5. Stir in stock and grated cauliflower.
6. Bring the mixture to a simmer and add cream.
7. Cook until liquid is reduced and cauliflower is al dente.
8. Serve warm and enjoy!

Nutritional info per serving:
Calories: 186 | Carbs: 6.7g | Fat: 16.5g | Protein: 2.8g

Zucchini Boats

The Zucchini Boats are filled with tomatoes, marinara sauce, Kalamata olives and others. They are full of nutrients and you will want more of them.
Prep time: 10 minutes | Cooking time: 25 minutes | Serving: 4

Ingredients:
- 3 cups chopped zucchini
- ½ cup marinara sauce
- ¼ red onion, sliced
- ¼ cup kalamata olives, chopped
- ½ cup cherry tomatoes, sliced
- 2 tablespoons fresh basil

Instructions:
1. Pre-heat your oven to 400°F.
2. Cut the zucchini half-lengthwise and shape them in boats.
3. Take a bowl and add tomato sauce, spread 1 layer of sauce on top of each of the boat.
4. Top with onion, olives, and tomatoes.
5. Bake for 20-25 minutes.
6. Top with basil and enjoy!

Nutritional info per serving:
Calories: 278 | Carbs: 10g | Fat: 20g | Protein: 15g

Roasted Onions and Green Beans

Roasted Onions and Green Beans are crunchy and can be ready in a short while. You can't go wrong with this recipe.
Prep time: 10 minutes | Cooking time: 15 minutes | Serving: 6

Ingredients:
- 1 yellow onion, sliced into rings
- ½ teaspoon onion powder
- 2 tablespoons coconut flour
- 1 1/3 pounds fresh green beans, trimmed and chopped

Instructions:
1. Take a large bowl and mix sunflower seeds with onion powder and coconut flour.
2. Add onion rings.
3. Mix well to coat.
4. Spread the rings in the baking sheet, lined with parchment paper.
5. Drizzle with some oil.
6. Bake for 10 minutes at 400°F.
7. Parboil the green beans for 3 to 5 minutes in the boiling water.
8. Drain and serve the beans with baked onion rings.
9. Serve warm and enjoy!

Nutritional info per serving:
Calories: 214 | Carbs:3.7g | Fat: 19.4g | Protein: 8.3g

Green Bean Roast

The green been roast is very fulfilling and ideal for eating as a dessert.
Prep time: 10 minutes | Cooking time: 20 minutes | Serving: 4

Ingredients:
- 1 whole egg
- 2 tablespoons olive oil
- Sunflower seeds and pepper to taste
- 1 pound fresh green beans
- 5 ½ tablespoons grated parmesan cheese

Instructions:
1. Pre-heat your oven to 400°F.
2. Take a bowl and whisk in eggs with oil and spices.
3. Add beans and mix well.
4. Stir in parmesan cheese and pour the mix into baking pan (lined with parchment paper.
5. Bake for 15-20 minutes. Serve warm and enjoy!

Nutritional info per serving:
Calories: 216 | Carbs: 7g | Fat: 21g | Protein: 9g

Almond and Blistered Beans

This recipe is so nice especially when crispy hot.
Prep time: 10 minutes | Cooking time: 20 minutes | Serving: 4

Ingredients:
- 1 pound fresh green beans, ends trimmed
- 1 ½ tablespoon olive oil
- ¼ teaspoon sunflower seeds
- 1 ½ tablespoons fresh dill, minced
- Juice of 1 lemon
- ¼ cup crushed almonds
- Sunflower seeds as needed

Instructions:
1. Pre-heat your oven to 400°F.
2. Add the green beans with your olive oil and also the sunflower seeds.
3. Then spread them in one single layer on a large sized sheet pan.
4. Roast it for 10 minutes and stir, then roast for another 8-10 minutes.
5. Remove from the oven and keep stirring in the lemon juice alongside the dill.
6. Top it with crushed almonds and some flaked sunflower seeds and serve.

Nutritional info per serving:
Calories: 347 | Carbs: 6g | Fat: 16g | Protein: 45g

Tomato Platter

This tomato platter will cheer your day and keep the hunger away from you.
Prep time: 10 minutes | Cooking time: - | Serving: 8

Ingredients:
- 1/3 cup olive oil
- 1 teaspoon sunflower seeds
- 2 tablespoons onion, chopped
- ¼ teaspoon pepper
- ½ a garlic, minced
- 1 tablespoon fresh parsley, minced
- 3 large fresh tomatoes, sliced
- 1 teaspoon dried basil
- ¼ cup red wine vinegar

Instructions:
1. Take a shallow dish and arrange tomatoes in the dish.
2. Add the rest of the ingredients in a mason jar, cover the jar and shake it well.
3. Pour the mix over tomato slices.
4. Let it chill for 2-3 hours.
5. Serve!

Nutritional info per serving:
Calories: 350 | Carbs: 10g | Fat: 28g | Protein: 14g

Lemony Sprouts

The lemony sprouts are yummy and easy to make. They are delicious and crispy.
Prep time: 10 minutes | Cooking time: 0 minutes | Serving: 4

Ingredients:
- 1 pound Brussels sprouts, trimmed and shredded
- 8 tablespoons olive oil
- 1 lemon, juice and zested
- Sunflower seeds and pepper to taste
- ¾ cup spicy almond and seed mix

Instructions:
1. Take a bowl and mix in lemon juice, sunflower seeds, pepper and olive oil.
2. Mix well.
3. Stir in shredded Brussels sprouts and toss.
4. Let it sit for 10 minutes.
5. Add nuts and toss.
6. Serve and enjoy!

Nutritional info per serving:
Calories: 382 | Carbs: 9g | Fat: 36g | Protein: 7g

Cauliflower Rice

Cauliflower rice is very nutritious and it will delight you as you eat. It is also very easy to prepare.

Prep time: 5 minutes | Cooking time: 6 minutes | Serving: 2

Ingredients:
- 1 head grated cauliflower head
- 1 tablespoon coconut aminos
- 1 pinch of sunflower seeds
- 1 pinch of black pepper
- 1 tablespoon Garlic Powder
- 1 tablespoon Sesame Oil

Instructions:
1. Add cauliflower to a food processor and grate it.
2. Take a pan and add sesame oil, let it heat up over medium heat.
3. Add grated cauliflower and pour coconut aminos.
4. Cook for 4-6 minutes.
5. Season and enjoy!

Nutritional info per serving:
Calories: 329 | Carbs: 13g | Fat: 28g | Protein: 10g

Chapter 5: Main Dishes

Stuffed Zucchini

This recipe will leave you satisfied as it is made to perfection.

Prep time: 5 minutes | Cooking time: 30 minutes | Servings: 2

Ingredients:
- 1 large zucchini
- 2 tbsp. olive oil
- ¼ cup green onion, chopped
- 1 garlic clove, minced
- 1 cup fresh baby spinach leaves
- A handful of fresh rocket, chopped
- Sea salt and black pepper to taste
- ¼ cup vegan cheese
- Pinch of dried parsley

Instructions:
1. Preheat oven to 380°F and use a parchment paper to line a baking tray.
2. Cut the zucchini in half lengthwise and scoop out most of the pulp.
3. Mash the zucchini pulp in a small bowl with a masher and set it aside.
4. Heat a skillet over medium heat and add half of the olive oil.
5. Add the zucchini pulp, chopped onion, and minced garlic to the skillet.
6. Stir continuously, cooking the ingredients for up to 5 minutes before adding the baby spinach and rocket.
7. Stir for a few seconds, add salt and pepper to taste, and turn off the heat.
8. Add the vegan cheese and stir well to ensure all ingredients are incorporated and the cheese has melted.
9. Scoop the mixture into the zucchini halves and transfer them onto the baking tray.
10. Cover the baking tray with aluminum foil and transfer it to the oven.
11. Bake the stuffed zucchini halves for 25 minutes. Then, turn off the oven, uncover the baking tray, and put the uncovered zucchini halves back into the oven for about 5 minutes.
12. Serve the stuffed zucchini garnished with the remaining olive oil and some dried parsley.
13. Serve and enjoy!

Nutritional info per serving:
Calories 359.5 | Carbs 7 g | Fats 32.5 g | Protein 7.3 g

Avocado Fries

These fries are easy to make and are incredibly tasty. Even if you are a picky eater, you will be impressed by this recipe!

Prep time: 3 minutes | Cooking time: 25 minutes | Servings: 2

Ingredients:
- 1 tbsp. olive oil
- ½ cup almond flour
- ¼ tsp. cayenne pepper
- ¼ tsp. smoked paprika
- Pinch of salt
- ¾ tbsp. unsweetened almond milk
- 1 medium Hass avocado, pitted, peeled
- 1 tsp. lime juice

Instructions:
1. Preheat the oven to 400°F.
2. Use a parchment paper to line a baking tray and grease the paper with olive oil.
3. In a small bowl, combine the flour, cayenne pepper, smoked paprika, and salt.
4. Pour the almond milk into another small bowl.
5. Slice the peeled avocado into 10 equally-sized fries.
6. Coat all sides of the fries in the flour mixture, dip in almond milk, and coat with another layer of flour.
7. Transfer the coated fries to the greased baking tray.
8. Bake the fries for 5 minutes, then flip them over and bake for another 10 minutes. Flip the fries again and bake for 5 more minutes.
9. Flip the fries one more time, sprinkle them with the lime juice, and bake them for a final 5 minutes.
10. Remove the baking tray out of the oven and allow the fries to cool down for a few minutes.
11. Serve warm with any low-carb (vegan) sauce and enjoy!

Nutritional info per serving:
Calories 333.7 | Carbs 4 g | Fats 31.9 g | Protein 7 g

Mushroom Zoodle Pasta

Is there anyone who does not like pasta? Unless you are allergic to them, you will love the Mushroom Zoodle Pasta.

Prep time: 10 minutes | Cooking time: 16 minutes | Servings: 4

Ingredients:
- 3 large zucchinis
- ½ tsp. salt
- 1 tbsp. coconut oil
- 1 large green onion, diced
- 3 garlic cloves, minced
- 5 cups oyster mushrooms, chopped
- Pinch each of nutmeg, onion powder, paprika powder, white pepper, and salt
- 1 cup full-fat coconut milk
- ½ cup vegan mozzarella
- ½ cup baby spinach leaves, chopped
- ¼ cup fresh thyme, chopped
- 1 tbsp. miso paste

Instructions:
1. In a large bowl, toss the zoodles or zucchini slices with half a teaspoon of salt and set aside.
2. Add coconut oil in a large skillet, over medium heat, and add the coconut oil.
3. Add the onion and cook until translucent, for about 5 minutes while stirring occasionally.
4. Stir in the minced garlic, chopped mushrooms, and remaining seasonings.
5. Cook all ingredients in the skillet for about 3 minutes, stirring continuously.
6. Reduce heat to medium-low and slowly incorporate the coconut milk, followed by the mozzarella.
7. Cover the skillet and let the ingredients heat through for about 8 minutes, stirring occasionally.
8. Drain any excess liquid from the salted zoodles by dabbing them with paper towels.
9. Add the dry zoodles to the skillet with the chopped spinach and stir well until all ingredients are combined.
10. Turn off the heat and top the mushroom zoodle pasta with the chopped thyme.
11. Add more seasonings to taste, serve the pasta in a bowl, and enjoy!

Nutritional info per serving:
Calories 421.6 | Carbs 13 g | Fats 34.9 g | Protein 11.5 g

Quick Veggie Protein Bowl

Whether it's for lunch or dinner, this recipe is ideal and will leave you wanting more.

Prep time: 5 minutes | Cooking time: 13 minutes | Servings: 1

Ingredients:
- 4 oz. extra-firm tofu, drained
- ¼ tsp. turmeric
- ¼ tsp. cayenne pepper
- 1 tbsp. coconut oil
- 1 cup broccoli florets, diced
- 1 cup Chinese kale, diced
- ½ cup button mushrooms, diced
- ½ tsp. dried oregano
- Himalayan salt
- Black pepper to taste
- ½ tsp. paprika
- ¼ cup of fresh oregano, diced

Instructions:
1. Cut the tofu into tiny pieces and season with the turmeric and cayenne pepper.
2. Warm a large skillet and add ¾ of the coconut oil.
3. Once oil is heated, add the tofu and cook it for about 5 minutes, stirring continuously.
4. Transfer the cooked tofu to a medium-sized bowl and set it aside.
5. Add the remaining coconut oil, diced broccoli florets, Chinese kale, button mushrooms, and the remaining herbs to the skillet. Use paprika, pepper, and salt to taste.
6. Cook the vegetables for 6-8 minutes, stirring continuously.
7. Transfer the cooked veggies and tofu to the bowl. Garnish with the optional fresh oregano.
8. Serve and enjoy!

Nutritional info per serving:
Calories 596 | Carbs 6 g | Fats 20.95 g | Protein 17.8 g

Vizza

This recipe is great a family dinner or a night out with your friends.

Prep time: minutes | Cooking time: minutes | Servings: 4

Ingredients:

Crust:
- 16 oz. cauliflower rice
- 3 flax eggs
- 2 tbsp. chia seeds
- ½ cup almond flour
- ½ tsp. garlic powder
- ½ tsp. dried basil
- Pinch of salt
- 2 tsp. water

Topping:
- ½ cup simple marinara sauce
- 1 medium zucchini, sliced
- 1 medium green bell pepper, pitted, cored, sliced
- 1 cup button mushrooms, diced
- ½ cup vegan cheese
- Sea salt
- Black pepper, ground
- 1 jalapeño pepper, pitted, cored, diced
- pinch of cayenne pepper
- A handful of fresh rockets

Instructions:
1. Preheat oven to 395°F and use a parchment paper to line a baking tray.
2. Transfer the cauliflower rice to a large saucepan and add enough water to cover the 'rice.' Over medium heat, bring the water to a soft boil. Cover the saucepan, turn down the heat to medium-low, and allow the rice to simmer for about 5 minutes before draining the water off. This step can be skipped if store-bought cauliflower rice is used.
3. Transfer the cauliflower rice onto a clean dish towel and close the cloth by holding the edges. Wring out any excess water by twisting the lower part of the towel that contains the rice.
4. Once the cauliflower rice is completely drained, transfer the towel to the freezer for up to 15 minutes. Doing so will cool the rice.
5. When the cauliflower rice has cooled completely, put it into a large bowl.
6. Add the flax eggs, chia seeds, almond flour, garlic, dried basil, and salt. Combine all the ingredients into a firm, kneadable dough. If the dough is too firm, add the optional 2 tablespoons of water.
7. Spread the dough over the baking dish's surface entire. The uncooked crust should be about ¼-inch thick.
8. Bake the crust in the oven for 25 minutes, then sprinkle some additional water on top and bake for another 5 minutes. The top of the crust will turn lightly golden.
9. Allow the crust to cool for a few minutes.
10. Spread the marinara sauce evenly over the golden crust. Do the same for the vegetables.
11. Finally, garnish the vizza with vegan cheese, optional jalapeño, and cayenne pepper.
12. Season the vizza with salt and pepper and transfer it back into the oven for a few more minutes.
13. Serve the vizza warm, garnished with a handful of fresh rocket, and enjoy!

Nutritional info per serving:
Calories 360.9 | Carbs 8 g | Fats 28.85 g | Protein 13.5 g

Tofu Cheese Nuggets & Zucchini Fries

Looking for a delicious recipe for a side dish, snack or an appetizer? This is it.

Prep time: 5 minutes | Cooking time: 18 minutes | Servings: 2

Ingredients:
Tofu Cheese Nuggets:
- 1 (12 oz. pack) extra-firm tofu, drained, cubed
- ½ cup smoked chipotle cream cheese
- ½ cup almond flour
- 2 tbsp. water

Zucchini Fries:
- 2 tsp. red chili flakes
- ½ cup almond flour
- ¼ cup olive oil
- 1 large zucchini, skinned

Instructions:
1. Preheat oven to 395°F and use a parchment paper to line a baking tray.
2. Put the cream cheese, ½ cup almond flour, and water into a large bowl and mix thoroughly until all the ingredients are combined.
3. Add in tofu cubes and coat all the cubes evenly.

4. Transfer the coated tofu cubes onto one half of the baking tray and set it aside.
5. Put the chili flakes and almond flour into a large bowl and mix until all ingredients are combined.
6. Pour the olive oil into a medium-sized bowl and dip each zucchini stick into the oil. Make sure to cover all fries evenly.
7. Put the zucchini fries in the bowl with the almond flour mixture and gently stir the fries around until they are all evenly covered.
8. Transfer the zucchini fries onto the baking tray with the tofu nuggets and spread them out evenly. If the nuggets and fries don't fit on the baking tray together, bake them in two batches.
9. Put the baking tray into the oven and bake the nuggets and fries for about 18 minutes, or until golden brown.
10. Allow the dish to cool down for about a minute.
11. Serve and enjoy with a light salad of greens as a side dish.

Nutritional info per serving:
Calories 813.5 | Carbs 7 g | Fats 72.1 g | Protein 30.35 g

Avocado Spring Rolls

These spring rolls are not just only for springtime, but can be enjoyed at any time during any season.
Prep time: 20 minutes | Cooking time: 1 minute | Servings: 4

Ingredients:
- 2 medium Hass avocados, peeled, pitted, sliced
- 1-inch piece ginger, grated
- 1 garlic clove, minced
- Juice of ½ lemon
- ½ cup cabbage, shredded
- ¼ cup carrots, julienned or matchsticks
- 4-6 coconut wraps
- 2 tbsp. olive oil

Spicy Almond Sauce:
- ½ cup almond butter
- 2 tsp. low-sodium soy sauce
- ½ tsp. rice vinegar
- Juice of ½ lemon
- ½ tsp. chili garlic paste
- 1 tbsp. low-carb maple syrup
- 2 tsp. sesame oil

Instructions:
1. Gently toss together the sliced avocado, ginger, garlic, lemon juice, cabbage, and julienned carrots in a small bowl.
2. Put a coconut wrap on a flat and dry surface. Place about ¼ of the avocado mixture in the center of the wrap.
3. Fold the wrap about ½ inch inward on two parallel sides and roll the wrap up until the mixture is covered.
4. Repeat with the remaining 3-5 wraps until all of the avocado mixture is used.
5. Put a skillet over medium-high heat and warm the olive oil until shimmering.
6. Add the spring rolls to the skillet and brown them, about 30 seconds on each side.
7. Put all the sauce ingredients into a medium-sized bowl and stir thoroughly. Add one or more tablespoons of warm water, if necessary, to achieve the desired consistency.
8. Serve the spring rolls warm with the spicy almond sauce as a dip and enjoy!

Nutritional info per serving:
Calories 503 | Carbs 11 g | Fats 45 g | Protein 10 g

Cauliflower Curry Soup

This keto Cauliflower Curry Soup is very nourishing and very healthy.
Prep time: 5 minutes | Cooking time: 40 minutes | Servings: 4

Ingredients:
- 1 large cauliflower, chopped
- 4 tbsp. olive oil
- ½ red onion, finely chopped
- 4 garlic cloves, minced
- 1 tbsp. yellow curry paste
- 1-inch piece ginger, grated
- 1 (12 oz. pack) extra-firm tofu, drained, scrambled
- 1 tsp. chili flakes
- Juice of 1 medium lime
- 4 cups vegetable broth
- 1 tbsp. sesame oil
- 1 tsp. low-sodium soy sauce
- 1 cup full-fat coconut milk

Instructions:
1. Preheat oven to 395°F and use a parchment paper to line a baking tray.

2. Put the cauliflower florets on the baking tray and drizzle 2 tablespoons of olive oil over them, covering them evenly.
3. Put the baking tray into the oven and bake for about 25-30 minutes, until the florets are golden brown.
4. Add the 2 tablespoons that remained of olive oil to a skillet over medium heat.
5. Remove the oven and put it aside for a few minutes to let the cauliflower florets cool down.
6. Add garlic and onion to the skillet and fry for about a minute, stirring occasionally.
7. Add the curry paste to the pot along with the ginger, scrambled tofu, and chili flakes. Stir for another minute.
8. Put the baked cauliflower florets into a blender or food processor, along with the vegetable broth, sesame oil, soy sauce, and coconut milk.
9. Blend these ingredients until smooth, then transfer the mixture into the pot.
10. Incorporate all the ingredients, occasionally stirring until the contents of the pot start to cook. Once the soup reaches the boiling point, bring the heat down to a simmer.
11. Cover and allow about 10 minutes to simmer. Take the pot the heat and set aside to cool for a few minutes.

Nutritional info per serving:
Calories 390.5 g | Carbs 6 g | Fats 34.2 g | Protein 12.25 g

Crispy Tofu Burgers

Burger is a favorite for many people. This recipe is crunchy and filled with flavor.
Prep time: 5 minutes | Cooking time: 20 minutes | Servings: 8

Ingredients:
- 10 oz. pack, drained extra-firm tofu
- 1 minced clove garlic
- ½ cup coconut milk
- 2 tbsp. soy sauce
- ¼ cup sesame oil
- 2 tbsp. rice vinegar
- 1 cup coconut flour

Crust:
- 1 tsp. chili flakes
- ¼ cup nori flakes
- ½ cup crushed cashews
- ½ cup sesame seeds

Instructions:
1. Preheat oven to 390°F and use a parchment paper to line on a baking tray.
2. Drain excess water from the tofu by press it on a plate. Slice into 8 and set aside.
3. Combine garlic, soy sauce, rice vinegar, coconut oil, and sesame oil in a medium-sized bowl.
4. In a different bowl, mix all ingredients of the crust.
5. In a third different bowl, add coconut flour and dip a tofu slice in the flour. To remove excess flour, shake it off.
6. Immerse the tofu in the mixture with coconut and then immerse it into the crust mix.
7. Put the tofu on the baking tray and repeat the process for the remainder of the tofu.
8. Space the tofu while on the baking tray.
9. Add the tofu to the oven and bake for 10 minutes on each side, or until crispy and brown.
10. Allow 2 minutes to cool before serving alongside a green salad.

Nutritional info per serving:
Calories 321 | Carbs 4 g | Fats 27.9 g | Protein 10.7 g

Baked Chicken Fajitas

This recipe is among the easiest that you can prepare. It has lots of flavor and there is no way you can fail to love this recipe.
Prep time: 10 minutes | Cooking Time: 18 minutes | Serve: 6

Ingredients:
- 1 1/2 lbs chicken tenders
- 2 tbsp fajita seasoning
- 2 tbsp olive oil
- 1 onion, sliced
- 2 bell pepper, sliced
- 1 lime juice
- 1 tsp kosher salt

Instructions:
1. Preheat the oven to 400 F.
2. Add all ingredients in a large mixing bowl and toss well.

3. Transfer bowl mixture on a baking tray and bake in preheated oven for 15-18 minutes.
4. Serve and enjoy.

Nutritional info per serving:
Calories 286 | Carbs 6.8 g | Fat 13 g | Protein 33 g

Baked Chicken Wings

Apart from the sweet flavor that it made of, this recipe takes less than an hour to be prepared and it is quite simple.

Prep time: 10 minutes | Cooking Time: 50 minutes | Serve: 4

Ingredients:
- 2 lbs chicken wings
- 1 tbsp. lemon pepper seasoning
- 2 tbsp butter, melted
- 4 tbsp olive oil

Instructions:
1. Preheat the oven to 400 F.
2. Toss chicken wings with olive oil.
3. Arrange chicken wings on a baking tray and bake for 50 minutes.
4. In a small bowl, mix together lemon pepper seasoning and butter.
5. Remove wings from oven and brush with butter and seasoning mixture.
6. Serve and enjoy.

Nutritional info per serving:
Calories 606 | Fat 36 g | Carbs 1 g | Sugar 0 g | Protein 65 g | Cholesterol 217 mg

Chicken with Spinach Broccoli

This recipe is so sweet that you might want to hide the left overs so that you can eat the following day!

Prep time: 10 minutes | Cooking Time: 10 minutes | Serve: 4

Ingredients:
- 1 lb chicken breasts, cut into pieces
- 4 oz cream cheese
- 1/2 cup parmesan cheese, shredded
- 2 cups baby spinach
- 2 cup broccoli florets
- 1 tomato, chopped
- 2 garlic cloves, minced
- 1 tsp Italian seasoning
- 2 tbsp olive oil
- Pepper
- Salt

Instructions:
1. Heat oil in a saucepan over medium-high heat.
2. Add chicken, season with pepper, Italian seasoning, and salt and sauté for 5 minutes or until chicken cooked through.
3. Add garlic and sauté for a minute.
4. Add cream cheese, parmesan cheese, spinach, broccoli, and tomato and cook for 3-4 minutes more.
5. Serve and enjoy.

Nutritional info per serving:
Calories 444 | Fat 28 g | Carbs 5.9 g | Protein 40 g

Delicious Bacon Chicken

This is roasted recipe and it has lots of flavors. It is also simple and easy to prepare. It is very awesomely delicious.

Prep time: 10 minutes | Cooking Time: 40 minutes | Serve: 6

Ingredients:
- 2 1/2 lbs chicken breasts, cut in half
- 4 oz cheddar cheese, shredded
- 1/2 lb bacon, cut into strips
- 1/2 tsp paprika
- 1/2 tsp onion powder
- 1/2 tsp garlic powder
- Pepper
- Salt

Instructions:
1. Preheat the oven to 400 F.
2. In a small bowl, mix together paprika, onion powder, garlic powder, pepper, and salt.
3. Rub chicken with spice mixture.
4. Place chicken on a baking tray and top each with bacon piece.
5. Bake for 30 minutes. Remove from oven and sprinkle with cheese and bake for 10 minutes more.
6. Serve and enjoy.

Nutritional info per serving:
Calories 642 | Fat 36 g | Carbs 1.2 g | Protein 73 g

Mexican Chicken

The Mexican Chicken recipe mouth-watering and so full of flavors!

Prep time: 10 minutes | Cooking Time: 25 minutes | Serve: 6

Ingredients:
- 2 cups chicken, cooked and shredded

- 1/2 cup Monterey jack cheese
- 1 1/2 cup cheddar cheese
- ¾ cup chicken broth
- 2 tsp taco seasoning
- 12 oz cauliflower rice
- 14 oz Rotel tomatoes
- 2 garlic cloves, minced
- 1/3 cup green pepper, diced
- 1 onion, diced
- 1 tbsp butter

Instructions:
1. Melt butter in a pan over medium heat.
2. Add garlic, pepper, and onion and sauté until softened.
3. Steam cauliflower rice according to packet instructions.
4. Add seasoning, broth, cauliflower rice, and Rotel to the pan.
5. Stir well and cook for 10 minutes.
6. Add chicken and cook for 5 minutes.
7. Top with cheese and cook until cheese is melted.
8. Serve and enjoy.

Nutritional info per serving:
Calories 270 | Fat 15 g | Carbs 8.1 g | Protein 24 g

Beef Casserole

The Beef Casserole is prepared in just half an hour! It is nourishing and very healthy.
Prep time: 10 minutes | Cooking Time: 35 minutes | Serve: 8

Ingredients:
- 1 lb ground beef
- ½ cup mozzarella cheese, shredded
- ½ cup cheddar cheese, shredded
- 2 cans green beans, drained
- ½ tsp garlic powder
- ½ cup heavy cream
- ½ cup chicken broth
- 3 oz cream cheese
- ½ tsp pepper
- ½ tsp salt

Instructions:
1. Preheat the oven to 350 F.
2. Brown meat in pan. Add cream cheese and stir until cheese is melted.
3. Add broth, garlic powder, heavy cream, pepper, and salt and stir well. Bring to boil.
4. Turn heat to medium and simmer until mixture thickened.
5. Add green beans then sprinkle cheese on top and bake in preheated oven for 25 minutes.
6. Serve and enjoy.

Nutritional info per serving:
Calories 280 | Carbs 4 g | Fat 20 g | Protein 18 g

Mexican Beef with Zucchini

You can never fail to love this delicious recipe. It is quickly prepared. It takes only 15 minutes to be prepared.
Prep time: 10 minutes | Cooking Time: 25 minutes | Serve: 6

Ingredients:
- 1 ½ lbs ground beef
- ¼ tsp red pepper flakes
- ½ tsp onion powder
- ½ tsp ground cumin
- ½ tbsp chili powder
- 10 oz salsa
- 2 garlic cloves, minced
- 2 zucchinis, diced
- ½ tsp pepper
- 1 tsp salt

Instructions:
1. Brown meat in pan with garlic, pepper, and salt.
2. Add tomatoes and spices and stir well.
3. Cover and simmer over low heat for 10 minutes.
4. Add remaining ingredients and cook for 10 minutes more.
5. Serve and enjoy.

Nutritional info per serving:
Calories 239 | Fat 7.5 g | Carbs 6.2 g | Protein 36 g

Mexican Beef

This recipe is combine the sweet taste of beef and the amazing taste of chili flakes, oregano and garlic which is such a delicious outcome.
Prep time: 10 minutes | Cooking Time: 9 Hours | Serve: 10

Ingredients:
- 3 lbs beef chuck roast
- ½ tsp red chili flakes
- 1 tsp dried oregano
- ½ tsp paprika
- 1 tsp cumin
- 1 tbsp chili powder

- 2 tbsp lemon juice
- 2 tbsp tomato paste
- 3 garlic cloves, minced
- 1 onion, diced
- 1 tsp kosher salt

Instructions:
1. In a small bowl, mix together all spices and set aside.
2. Add onion, garlic, lemon juice, and tomato paste in slow cooker and stir well.
3. Place meat into the slow cooker and sprinkle spice mixture all over meat.
4. Cover and cook on low for 8 hours.
5. Remove meat from slow cooker and shred using fork.
6. Return shredded meat to the slow cooker and cook for 60 minutes more.
7. Serve and enjoy.

Nutritional info per serving:
Calories 507 | Fat 38 g | Carbs 2.7 g | Protein 36 g

Asian Beef Stew

The recipe is finger licking sweet. It is also keto friendly!
Prep time: 10 minutes | Cooking Time: 5 hours 15 minutes | Serve: 8

Ingredients:
- 3 lbs beef stew meat, trimmed
- 2 tsp ginger, minced
- 2 garlic cloves, minced
- 1/3 cup tomato paste
- 14.5 oz can coconut milk
- 1 medium onion, sliced
- 2 tbsp olive oil
- 2 cups carrots, julienned
- 2 cups broccoli florets
- 2 tsp fresh lime juice
- 2 tbsp soy sauce
- 1/2 cup curry paste
- 2 Tsp sea salt

Instructions:
1. Heat 1 tbsp oil in a pan over medium-high heat.
2. Add meat and brown the meat on all sides.
3. Transfer meat to crock pot.
4. Add remaining oil in a pan and sauté ginger, garlic, and onion over medium-high heat for 5 minutes.
5. Add coconut milk and stir well.
6. Transfer pan mixture to the crock pot.
7. Add remaining ingredients except for carrots and broccoli into the crock pot.
8. Cover and cook on high for 5 hours.
9. Add carrots and broccoli during the last 30 minutes of cooking.
10. Serve and enjoy.

Nutritional info per serving:
Calories 535 | Fat 28 g | Carbs 12 g | Protein 55 g

Beef Roast

If you are looking a perfect roasted meat, then this is the right one. It is easy to prepare but takes 5 hours. It is worth the wait.
Prep time: 10 minutes | Cooking Time: 5 Hours | Serve: 6

Ingredients:
- 2 1/2 lbs beef roast
- 1 tbsp ground coriander
- 1 tbsp garam masala
- 1 Serrano pepper, minced
- 1 tbsp ginger, grated
- 5 garlic cloves, minced
- 2 tbsp fresh lemon juice
- 20 curry leaves
- 1 tsp mustard seeds
- 2 tbsp coconut oil
- 1 large onion, chopped
- 1/4 cup coconut slices
- 1/2 tsp ground pepper
- 1 tsp turmeric
- 1 1/2 tsp chili powder
- 1 tsp salt

Instructions:
1. Add oil, mustard seeds, onion, and salt into the crock pot and cook on high for 1 hour.
2. Add remaining ingredients except for coconut and cook on high for 3 hours.
3. Shred meat using a fork.
4. Add coconut slices and cook on high for 1 hour.
5. Serve and enjoy.

Nutritional info per serving:
Calories 445 | Fat 19 g | Carbs 7 g | Protein 59 g

Almond Cinnamon Beef Meatballs

Meatballs are loved by most people that eat meat and therefore this is no exception.
Prep time: 10 minutes | Cooking Time: 25 minutes | Serve: 8

Ingredients:
- 2 lbs ground beef
- 3 eggs
- ½ cup fresh parsley, minced
- 1 tsp cinnamon
- 1 ½ tsp dried oregano
- 2 tsp cumin
- 1 tsp garlic, minced
- 1 cup almond flour
- 1 medium onion, grated
- 1 tsp pepper
- 2 tsp salt

Instructions:
1. Preheat the oven to 400 F.
2. Add all ingredients into the mixing bowl and mix until well combined.
3. Make small meatballs from mixture and place on greased baking tray and bake for 20-25 minutes.
4. Serve and enjoy.

Nutritional info per serving:
Calories 325 | Fat 16 g | Carbs 6 g | Protein 40 g

Creamy Beef Stroganoff

It is keto friendly and its ingredients are healthy. It takes 40 minutes to get this spicy recipe ready!
Prep time: 10 minutes | Cooking Time: 20 minutes | Serve: 4

Ingredients:
- 1 lb beef strips
- 3/4 cup mushrooms, sliced
- 1 small onion, chopped
- 1 tbsp butter
- 2 tbsp olive oil
- 2 tbsp green onion, chopped
- 1/4 cup sour cream
- 1 cup chicken broth
- Pepper
- Salt

Instructions:
1. Add meat in bowl and coat with 1 teaspoon oil, pepper and salt.
2. Heat remaining oil in a pan.
3. Add meat to pan and cook until golden brown on both sides.
4. Transfer meat in bowl and set aside.
5. Add butter in same pan.
6. Add onion and cook until onion softened.
7. Add mushrooms and sauté until the liquid is absorbed.
8. Add broth and cook until sauce thickened.
9. Add sour cream, green onion, and meat and stir well.
10. Cook over medium-high heat for 3-4 minutes.
11. Serve and enjoy.

Nutritional info per serving:
Calories 345 | Fat 20 g | Carbs 3 g | Protein 35 g

Buttery Lamb Chops

The Buttery Lamb Chops are filled with lots of flavor. They are not too spicy and therefore ideal even to little kids. They are one the perfect recipes for holidays.
Prep time: 10 minutes | Cooking Time: 10 minutes | Serve: 4

Ingredients:
- 1 lb lamb chops
- 2 garlic cloves, minced
- 2 tbsp fresh basil, chopped
- 1/2 tsp garlic powder
- 2 tbsp butter
- 1 1/2 tsp Dijon mustard
- 1 tbsp olive oil

Instructions:
1. Season pork chops with garlic powder and brush with oil.
2. Heat grill over medium-high heat.
3. Cook pork chops on hot grill for 4-5 minutes per side.
4. In a small bowl, mix together butter, mustard, and basil.
5. Spread butter mixture on each pork chops and Servings.

Nutritional info per serving:
Calories 295 | Fat 17.6 g | Carbs 0.6 g | Protein 32.1 g

Lemon Herb Lamb Chops

They are seared to form a herb and garlic crust which makes it even more amazing. The cooking time is very little after you have prepared everything; just 10 minutes!
Prep time: 10 minutes | Cooking Time: 10 minutes | Serve: 4

Ingredients:
- 1 1/2 lbs lamb chops
- 1/4 cup olive oil

- 1/4 tsp pepper
- 1 1/2 tsp oregano
- 1 tsp thyme
- 2 garlic cloves, chopped
- 2 tbsp lemon juice
- 1/4 tsp salt

Instructions:
1. Marinate the lamb chops in the mixture of garlic, oregano, thyme, lemon juice, olive oil, pepper, and salt. Cover and place in the fridge overnight.
2. Cook pork chops over a hot grill for 3-5 minutes per side.
3. Serve and enjoy.

Nutritional info per serving:
Calories 435 | Fat 24 g | Carbs 2 g | Protein 48 g

Fennel Grill Pork Chops

You will want to have more of this recipe because of its deliciousness! It is keto compliant

Prep time: 10 minutes | Cooking Time: 10 minutes | Serve: 4

Ingredients:
- 4 pork chops, bone-in
- 1 ¾ tsp dried sage, crumbled
- 1 tsp fennel seed, crushed
- 1/2 tsp dried thyme
- 1 ½ tsp dried rosemary, crumbled
- 1/3 cup olive oil
- 1 bay leaf, crushed
- 1 ½ tsp salt

Instructions:
1. In a bowl, mix together sage, bay leaf, fennel seed, thyme, rosemary, and salt.
2. Rub pork chops with herb sage mixture and brush with olive oil and place in fridge for overnight.
3. Preheat the grill over medium heat.
4. Place marinated pork chops on the hot grill and cook for 4 minutes on each side.
5. Serve and enjoy.

Nutritional info per serving:
Calories 404 | Fat 37 g | Carbs 1 g

Herb Pork Roast

This Herb Pork Roast recipe is perfectly roasted to bring out the sweet flavors and healthy nutrients in its ingredients.

Prep time: 10 minutes | Cooking Time: 1 Hour | Serve: 6

Ingredients:
- 4 lbs pork loin roast, boneless
- 1/4 cup fresh sage leaves
- 1/3 cup fresh rosemary leaves
- 2 garlic cloves, peeled
- ¼ cup lemon juice
- ¼ tsp pepper
- 1/2 tbsp salt

Instructions:
1. Add sage, rosemary, garlic, lemon juice, pepper, and salt into the blender and blend until smooth.
2. Rub herb paste over roast and place on hot grill.
3. Close grill hood and cook for 1 hour.
4. Sliced and serve.

Nutritional info per serving:
Calories 655 | Fat 30 g | Carbs 4 g | Protein 87 g

Asian Pork Hock

It is filled with lots of flavor and healthy fats and the texture is just right.

Prep time: 10 minutes | Cooking Time: 4 Hours | Serve: 2

Ingredients:
- 1 lb pork hock
- 2 garlic cloves, crushed
- ½ tsp oregano
- ½ tsp Chinese five spice
- 1 tbsp butter
- 1 onion, sliced
- ¼ cup erythritol
- 1/3 cup white wine
- 1/3 cup soy sauce
- ¼ cup rice vinegar

Instructions:
1. Spray pan with cooking spray and heat over medium heat.
2. Add onion and sauté until soften.
3. Transfer onion in crock pot.
4. Browned meat in same pan from all sides.
5. Transfer meat in crock pot along with remaining ingredients and cook for 2 hours.
6. Stir well and cook for 2 hours more.
7. Serve and enjoy.

Nutritional info per serving:

Calories 321 | Fat 14.9 g | Carbs 5.5 g | Protein 33.8 g

Parmesan Meatballs

If you do not love meatballs, it is most likely that you haven't tried these ones yet.
Prep time: 10 minutes | Cooking Time: 20 minutes | Serve: 12

Ingredients:
- 1 lb ground beef
- 1 egg
- ¼ cup parmesan cheese, shredded
- ¼ cup fresh parsley, chopped
- 1 tsp Italian seasoning
- ½ tsp garlic powder
- 2 tbsp onion, chopped
- 1/3 cup coconut milk
- ½ cup breadcrumbs
- 1 lb ground pork
- Pepper
- Salt

Instructions:
1. Preheat the oven to 400 F.
2. Add all ingredients into the large bowl and mix until well combined.
3. Make balls from meat mixture and place on greased baking tray.
4. Bake for 20 minutes.
5. Serve and enjoy.

Nutritional info per serving:
Calories 193 | Fat 7 g | Carbs 4.3 g | Protein 25 g

Beef Shawarma

They have low calories and are high in flavors and above all, they are keto friendly! Isn't that awesome? It definitely is. So, try it today!
Prep time: 10 minutes | Cooking Time: 15 minutes | Serve: 4

Ingredients:
- 1 lb ground beef
- ¼ cup parsley, chopped
- 3 cups cabbage, shredded
- 1 cup onion, sliced
- 2 tbsp olive oil
- 2 tbsp shawarma mix
- 1 tsp salt

Instructions:
1. Heat oil in a pan over medium-high heat.
2. Add meat to the pan and cook until meat is no longer pink.
3. Add onion and sauté onion for 3-4 minutes.
4. Add shawarma mix and salt and stir well.
5. Add cabbage and stir to combine.
6. Add 2 tbsp water and cook for 1 minute.
7. Garnish with parsley and serve.

Nutritional info per serving:
Calories 152 | Fat 12 g | Carbs 7 g | Protein 25 g

Shrimp and Broccoli

This comforting Shrimp and Broccoli is a keto recipe that has nice flavors!
Prep time: 10 minutes | Cooking Time: 7 minutes | Serve: 2

Ingredients:
- 1/2 lb shrimp
- 1 tsp fresh lemon juice
- 2 tbsp butter
- 2 garlic cloves, minced
- 1 cup broccoli florets
- Salt

Instructions:
1. Melt butter in a pan over medium heat.
2. Add garlic and broccoli to pan and cook for 3-4 minutes.
3. Add shrimp and cook for 3-4 minutes.
4. Add lemon juice and salt and stir well.
5. Serve and enjoy.

Nutritional info per serving:
Calories 257 | Fat 13 g | Carbs 6 g | Protein 27 g

Baked Salmon

If you are looking a perfect seafood, then this is the right one
Prep time: 10 minutes | Cooking Time: 35 minutes | Serve: 4

Ingredients:
- 1 lb salmon fillet
- 4 tbsp parsley, chopped
- 1/4 cup mayonnaise
- 1/4 cup parmesan cheese, grated
- 2 garlic cloves, minced
- 2 tbsp butter

Instructions:
1. Preheat the oven to 350 F.
2. Place salmon on greased baking tray.
3. Melt butter in a pan over medium heat.
4. Add garlic and sauté for minute.
5. Add remaining ingredient and stir to combined.

6. Spread pan mixture over salmon fillet.
7. Bake for 20-25 minutes.
8. Serve and enjoy.

Nutritional info per serving:
Calories 412 | Fat 26 g | Carbs 4.3 g | Protein 34 g

Buttery Shrimp

Wondering on what to serve for the next homemade brunch? Wonder no more because this is the perfect recipe that!
Prep time: 5 minutes | Cooking Time: 15 minutes | Serve: 4

Ingredients:
- 1 1/2 lbs shrimp
- 1 tbsp Italian seasoning
- 1 lemon, sliced
- 1 stick butter, melted

Instructions:
1. Add all ingredients into the large mixing bowl and toss well.
2. Transfer shrimp mixture on baking tray.
3. Bake at 350 F for 15 minutes.
4. Serve and enjoy.

Nutritional info per serving:
Calories 415 | Fat 26 g | Carbs 3 g | Protein 39 g

Avocado Shrimp Salad

Who doesn't love salad? It can be ready in a matter of few minutes.
Prep time: 10 minutes | Cooking Time: 10 minutes | Serve: 6

Ingredients:
- 1 lb shrimp
- 3 bacon slices, cooked and crumbled
- 1/4 cup feta cheese, crumbled
- 1 tbsp lemon juice
- 1/2 cup tomatoes, chopped
- 2 avocados, chopped
- 2 garlic cloves, minced
- 1 tbsp olive oil
- Pepper
- Salt

Instructions:
1. Heat oil in a pan over medium heat.
2. Add garlic and sauté for minute.
3. Add shrimp, pepper, and salt and cook for 5-7 minutes. Remove from heat and set aside.
4. Meanwhile, add remaining ingredients to the large mixing bowl.

5. Add shrimp and toss well.
6. Cover and place in fridge for 1 hour.
7. Serve and enjoy.

Nutritional info per serving:
Calories 268 | Fat 18 g | Carbs 8.1 g | Protein 19.6 g

Shrimp and Garlic

The combination of Shrimp and Garlic will definitely leave you wanting more.
Prep time: 5 minutes | Cooking Time: 15 minutes | Serve: 4

Ingredients:
- 1 lb shrimp, peeled and deveined
- 1 tsp parsley, chopped
- 2 tbsp lemon juice
- 5 garlic cloves, minced
- 3 tbsp butter
- Salt

Instructions:
1. Melt butter in a pan over high heat.
2. Add shrimp in pan and cook for 1 minutes. Season with salt.
3. Stir and cook shrimp until turn to pink.
4. Add lemon juice and garlic and cook for 2 minutes.
5. Turn heat to medium and cook for 4 minutes more.
6. Garnish with parsley and serve.

Nutritional info per serving:
Calories 219 | Fat 10.6 g | Carbs 3.2 g | Protein 26 g

Salmon Patties

This recipe is so sweet. It brings in the best things as concerns salmon.
Prep time: 10 minutes | Cooking Time: 10 minutes | Serve: 3

Ingredients:
- 14.5 oz can salmon
- 4 tbsp butter
- 1 avocado, diced
- 2 eggs, lightly beaten
- 1/2 cup almond flour
- 1/2 onion, minced
- Pepper
- Salt

Instructions:
1. Add all ingredients except butter in a large mixing bowl and mix until well combined.

2. Make six patties from mixture. Set aside.
3. Melt butter in a pan over medium heat.
4. Place patties on pan and cook for 4-5 minutes on each side.
5. Serve and enjoy.

Nutritional info per serving:
Calories 619 | Fat 49 g | Carbs 11 g | Protein 36 g

Tuna Salad

This salad is so tasty! Do not wait any longer as you can prepare this recipe as soon as today!

Prep time: 5 minutes | Cooking Time: 5 minutes | Serve: 2

Ingredients:
- 5 oz can tuna, drained
- 1 tsp Dijon mustard
- 2 tbsp dill pickles, chopped
- 1 tbsp fresh chives, chopped
- 2 tbsp mayonnaise
- Pepper
- Salt

Instructions:
1. Add all ingredients into the large bowl and mix well.
2. Serve and enjoy.

Nutritional info per serving:
Calories 143 | Fat 5.6 g | Carbs 4 g | Protein 18 g

Shrimp Scampi

It is also simple and easy to prepare. It is very awesomely delicious.

Prep time: 10 minutes | Cooking Time: 25 minutes | Serve: 4

Ingredients:
- 1 lb shrimp, peeled and deveined
- 4 tbsp parmesan cheese, grated
- 1 cup chicken broth
- 1 tbsp garlic, minced
- 1/2 cup butter

Instructions:
1. Preheat the oven to 350 F.
2. Melt butter in a saucepan over medium heat.
3. Add garlic and sauté for minute. Add broth and stir well.
4. Add shrimp to glass dish and pour butter mixture over shrimp.
5. Top with grated cheese and bake for 10-12 minutes.

6. Serve and enjoy.

Nutritional info per serving:
Calories 388 | Fat 27 g | Carbs 2.7 g | Protein 30.4 g

Grilled Salmon

The pepper and garlic make the recipe mouth-watering and so full of flavors!

Prep time: 10 minutes | Cooking Time: 25 minutes | Serve: 4

Ingredients:
- 4 salmon fillets
- 1 tsp dried rosemary
- 3 garlic cloves, minced
- 1/4 tsp pepper
- 1 tsp salt

Instructions:
1. In a bowl, mix together rosemary, garlic, pepper, and salt.
2. Add salmon fillets in a bowl and coat well and let sit for 15 minutes.
3. Preheat the grill.
4. Place marinated salmon fillets on hot grill and cook for 10-12 minutes.
5. Serve and enjoy.

Nutritional info per serving:
Calories 240 | Fat 11 g | Carbs 1 g | Protein 34 g

Salmon with Sauce

Salmon with Sauce could be the best baked seafood that you could taste in a very long time!

Prep time: 10 minutes | Cooking Time: 3 minutes | Serve: 4

Ingredients:
- 1 lb salmon
- 1/2 lemon juice
- 1 tbsp garlic, minced
- 1 tbsp Dijon mustard
- 1 tbsp dill, chopped
- 1 tbsp mayonnaise
- 1/3 cup sour cream
- Pepper
- Salt

Instructions:
1. Preheat the oven to 425 F.
2. In a bowl, mix together sour cream, lemon juice, dill, Dijon, and mayonnaise.
3. Place salmon on baking tray and top with garlic, pepper, and salt.

4. Pour half sour cream mixture over salmon.
5. Cover and bake for 20 minutes. Uncover and bake for 10 minutes more.
6. Serve with remaining sauce.

Nutritional info per serving:
Calories 213 | Fat 12 g | Carbs 3.1 g | Sugar 0.3 g | Protein 23 g

Parmesan Salmon

The combination of the salmon fillets and parmesan will definitely leave you wanting more.

Prep time: 10 minutes | Cooking Time: 15 minutes | Serve: 5

Ingredients:
- 1 1/2 lbs salmon fillets
- 1 tsp BBQ seasoning
- 1 tsp paprika
- 1 tbsp olive oil
- 4 tbsp parsley, chopped
- 3 garlic cloves, minced
- 1/2 cup parmesan cheese, shredded
- Pepper
- Salt

Instructions:
1. Preheat the oven to 425 F.
2. Drizzle oil over salmon and sprinkle with seasonings.
3. In a small bowl, mix together parsley, cheese, and garlic and sprinkle on top of salmon.
4. Place salmon to a baking tray and cover with parchment paprt.
5. Bake for 10 minutes. Uncover and bake for 5 minutes more.
6. Serve and enjoy.

Nutritional info per serving:
Calories 209 | Fat 11 g | Carbs 1 g | Sugar 0.1 g | Protein 26 g

Shrimp Stir Fry

This recipe has low calories and are high in flavors and above all, they are easy to make!

Prep time: 10 minutes | Cooking Time: 15 minutes | Serve: 4

Ingredients:
- 8 shrimp, peeled
- 1 tbsp parsley, chopped
- 2 tsp red pepper flakes
- 1 tsp garlic, minced
- 1 cup cabbage, shredded
- 1/4 cup water
- 2 1/2 tbsp butter

Instructions:
1. Melt 1 tbsp butter in a pan over high heat.
2. Add cabbage and 1 tbsp water and stir for 1 minute.
3. Transfer cabbage on a plate.
4. Melt remaining butter in same pan.
5. Add shrimp and garlic and cook until shrimp turns to pink.
6. Add remaining ingredients and cook for 1 minute.
7. Pour pan mixture over cabbage and serve.

Nutritional info per serving:
Calories 125 | Fat 8 g | Carbs 2.5 g | Protein 10 g

Zucchini Eggplant with Cheese

It is a perfect recipe to make for your guests and family. It takes little time to have this aromatic recipe ready.

Prep time: 10 minutes | Cooking Time: 40 minutes | Serve: 6

Ingredients:
- 1 medium eggplant, sliced
- 4 tbsp parsley, chopped
- ½ cup fresh basil, chopped
- 3 zucchinis, sliced
- 3 oz Parmesan cheese, grated
- 1 tbsp olive oil
- 1 cup cherry tomatoes, cut in half
- 2 garlic cloves, minced
- 1/4 tsp pepper
- 1/4 tsp salt

Instructions:
1. Preheat the oven to 350 F.
2. In a bowl, add cherry tomatoes, eggplant, zucchini, olive oil, garlic, cheese, basil, pepper and salt toss well.
3. Transfer the eggplant mixture into the baking dish and bake for 35 minutes.
4. Garnish with chopped parsley and serve.

Nutritional info per serving:
Calories 111 | Fat 6 g | Carbs 11 g | Protein 7 g

Turnips Mashed

This keto friendly mashed turnips is so tasty and full of flavors that you will want to make it again!

Prep time: 10 minutes | Cooking Time: 10 minutes | Serve: 4

Ingredients:
- 3 cups turnip, diced
- 3 tbsp butter, melted
- 1/4 cup heavy cream
- 2 garlic cloves, minced
- ¼ tsp garlic powder
- ¼ tsp onion powder
- Pepper
- Salt

Instructions:
1. Boil turnips in a saucepan until tender. Drain well and mashed turnips until smooth.
2. Add remaining ingredients and mix well.
3. Serve and enjoy.

Nutritional info per serving:
Calories 130 | Fat 12 g | Carbs 7 g | Protein 2 g

Coconut Cauliflower Rice

It does not take much time when making it. It takes only 7 minutes. You will absolutely love this amazing recipe!

Prep time: 10 minutes | Cooking Time: 7 minutes | Serve: 2

Ingredients:
- 2 cups cauliflower, chopped
- 2 tbsp water
- 2 tbsp unsweetened shredded coconut
- 2 tbsp coconut oil
- 1 tsp lime zest
- 1 tbsp fresh cilantro, chopped
- 3 tbsp coconut milk powder

Instructions:
1. Add cauliflower, water, shredded coconut, coconut oil, and coconut milk powder in a microwave-safe dish and microwave on high for 7 minutes.
2. Add lime zest and cilantro and stir well.
3. Serve and enjoy.

Nutritional info per serving:
Calories 195 | Fat 19 g | Carbs 6 g | Protein 2 g

Parmesan Zucchini Chips

This easy recipe can be prepared even after a long day at work because it takes a few minutes.

Prep time: 10 minutes | Cooking Time: 15 minutes | Serve: 3

Ingredients:
- 2 medium zucchinis, sliced
- ½ tsp garlic powder
- ¼ tsp onion powder
- 1/2 cup parmesan cheese, grated
- Pepper
- Salt

Instructions:
1. Arrange sliced zucchinis on a baking tray. Season with garlic powder, onion powder, pepper, and salt.
2. Sprinkle parmesan cheese on top of zucchini slices.
3. Bake at 425 F for 15 minutes.
4. Serve and enjoy.

Nutritional info per serving:
Calories 45 | Fat 2 g | Carbs 6 g | Protein 4 g

Olive Cheese Omelet

Apart from tasting good, this recipe also looks beautiful. It is keto compliant

Prep time: 10 minutes | Cooking Time: 5 minutes | Serve: 4

Ingredients:
- 4 large eggs
- 2 oz cheese
- 12 olives, pitted
- 2 tbsp butter
- 2 tbsp olive oil
- 1 tsp herb de Provence
- 1/2 tsp salt

Instructions:
1. Add all ingredients except butter in a bowl whisk well until frothy.
2. Melt butter in a pan over medium heat.
3. Pour egg mixture onto hot pan and spread evenly.
4. Cover and cook for 3 minutes.
5. Turn omelet to other side and cook for 2 minutes more.
6. Serve and enjoy.

Nutritional info per serving:
Calories 250 | Fat 23 g | Carbs 2 g | Protein 10 g

Cheese Almond Pancakes

This recipe is packed with ingredients which are a good source of nutrients and vitamins!

Prep time: 10 minutes | Cooking Time: 10 minutes | Serve: 4

Ingredients:
- 4 eggs
- 1/4 tsp cinnamon

- 1/2 cup cream cheese
- 1/2 cup almond flour
- 1 tbsp butter, melted

Instructions:
1. Add all ingredients into the blender and blend until combined.
2. Melt butter in a pan over medium heat.
3. Pour 3 tablespoons of batter per pancake and cook for 2 minutes on each side.
4. Serve and enjoy.

Nutritional info per serving:
Calories 271 | Fat 25 g | Carbs 5 g | Protein 10.8 g

Cauliflower Frittata

It is a very healthy meal that is good for a large family.
Prep time: 10 minutes | Cooking Time: 5 minutes | Serve: 1

Ingredients:
- 1 egg
- 1/2 tbsp onion, diced
- ¼ cup cauliflower rice
- 1 tbsp olive oil
- 1/4 tsp turmeric
- Pepper
- Salt

Instructions:
1. Add all ingredients except oil into the bowl and mix well to combine.
2. Heat oil in a pan over medium heat.
3. Pour the mixture into the hot oil pan and cook for 3-4 minutes.
4. Serve and enjoy.

Nutritional info per serving:
Calories 196 | Fat 19 g | Carbs 3 g | Protein 7 g

Basil Tomato Frittata

It one of the healthy recipes that we have around and therefore highly recommended for everyone.
Prep time: 10 minutes | Cooking Time: 15 minutes | Serve: 2

Ingredients:
- 5 eggs
- 1 tbsp olive oil
- 7 oz can artichokes
- 1 garlic clove, chopped
- 1 onion, chopped
- 1/2 cup cherry tomatoes
- 2 tbsp fresh basil, chopped
- 1/4 cup feta cheese, crumbled
- 1/4 tsp pepper
- 1/4 tsp salt

Instructions:
1. Heat oil in a pan over medium heat.
2. Add garlic and onion and sauté for 4 minutes.
3. Add artichokes, basil, and tomatoes and cook for 4 minutes.
4. Beat eggs in a bowl and season with pepper and salt.
5. Pour egg mixture into the pan and cook for 5-7 minutes.
6. Serve and enjoy.

Nutritional info per serving:
Calories 325 | Fat 22 g | Carbs 14 g | Sugar 6.2 g | Protein 20 g

Chia Spinach Pancakes

This recipe is loaded with lots of nutrition and flavor which is ideal for whole family or for any occasion!
Prep time: 10 minutes | Cooking Time: 5 minutes | Serve: 6

Ingredients:
- 4 eggs
- ½ cup coconut flour
- 1 cup coconut milk
- ¼ cup chia seeds
- 1 cup spinach, chopped
- 1 tsp baking soda
- ½ tsp pepper
- ½ tsp salt

Instructions:
1. Whisk eggs in a bowl until frothy.
2. Combine together all dry ingredients and add in egg mixture and whisk until smooth. Add spinach and stir well.
3. Greased pan with butter and heat over medium heat.
4. Pour 3-4 tablespoons of batter onto the pan and make pancake.
5. Cook pancake until lightly golden brown from both the sides.
6. Serve and enjoy.

Nutritional info per serving:
Calories 111 | Fat 7.2 g | Carbs 6 g | Protein 6.3 g

Feta Kale Frittata

This keto friendly recipe is a very simple recipe to make! It is also rich in fresh flavors that make eaters want more of it!

Prep time: 10 minutes | Cooking Time: 2 Hour 10 minutes | Serve: 8

Ingredients:
- 8 eggs, beaten
- 4 oz feta cheese, crumbled
- 6 oz bell pepper, roasted and diced
- 5 oz baby kale
- 1/4 cup green onion, sliced
- 2 tsp olive oil

Instructions:
1. Heat olive oil in a pan over medium-high heat.
2. Add kale to the pan and sauté for 4-5 minutes or until softened.
3. Spray slow cooker with cooking spray.
4. Add cooked kale into the slow cooker.
5. Add green onion and bell pepper into the slow cooker.
6. Pour beaten eggs into the slow cooker and stir well to combine.
7. Sprinkle crumbled feta cheese.
8. Cook on low for 2 hours or until frittata is set.
9. Serve and enjoy.

Nutritional info per serving:
Calories 150 | Fat 9 g | Carbs 10 g | Protein 10 g

Protein Muffins

The Sesame Chicken recipe has ingredients that are full of nutrients such as proteins and vitamins.

Prep time: 10 minutes | Cooking Time: 15 minutes | Serve: 12

Ingredients:
- 8 eggs
- 2 scoop vanilla protein powder
- 8 oz cream cheese
- 4 tbsp butter, melted

Instructions:
1. In a large bowl, combine together cream cheese and melted butter.
2. Add eggs and protein powder and whisk until well combined.
3. Pour batter into the greased muffin pan.
4. Bake at 350 F for 25 minutes.
5. Serve and enjoy.

Nutritional info per serving:
Calories 149 | Fat 12 g | Carbs 2 g | Protein 8 g

Chapter 6: Breads & Rolls

Low-carb dinner rolls

These dinner rolls are the best and very easy to make, delicious and filling. Try them today.
Prep time: 10 minutes | Cooking time: 10 minutes | Servings 6

Ingredients
- 1 cup almond flour
- ¼ cup flaxseed (ground)
- 1 cup Mozzarella (shredded)
- 1 oz cream cheese
- ½ tsp baking soda
- 1 egg

Instructions:
1. Preheat your oven to 400°F.
2. Using a microwave-safe mixing bowl, put both the mozzarella and cream cheese. Microwave it for one minute. Stir them till they become smooth.
3. Add eggs in the bowl and stir till they mix well.
4. In another clean bowl, put your flaxseed, almond flour and baking soda and mix the dry ingredients.
5. Pour your egg and cheese mix into the bowl with dry ingredients. Use your hand mixer or hands to make dough by kneading.
6. Slightly wet your hands with coconut oil or olive oil and roll your dough to six balls.
7. Top them with sesame seeds and place them on the parchment paper.
8. Bake them for 10 minutes. A golden brown look will indicate that they are done.
9. Leave them to cool.

Nutritional info per serving:
Calories: 218 | Carbs: 5.6g | Fat: 18g | Protein: 10.7g

Low-carb clover rolls

They are gluten free, fluffy, cheesy and soft.
Prep time: 10 minutes | Cooking time: 20 minutes | Servings 8

Ingredients
- 1/3 cup coconut flour or 1 1/3 cup almond flour
- 1 ½ cup mozzarella cheese (shredded)
- 1 ½ tsp baking powder
- ¼ cup parmesan cheese (grated)
- 2 ounces cream cheese
- 2 eggs (large)

Instructions:
1. Preheat your oven to 350°F.
2. Put your almond flour and baking powder in a clean bowl and mix.
3. Using another bowl, put your Mozzarella and cream cheese and microwave for a minute. Stir it well after it melts.
4. Add eggs to the cheese and stir.
5. Add the egg-cheese mix to the bowl with dry ingredients and mix thoroughly.
6. Wet your hands and knead dough into a sticky ball.
7. Put the dough ball on the parchment paper and slice into fourths.
8. Slice each fourth or quarter into 6 smaller portions.
9. Roll each small portion into balls.
10. Roll the balls into the parmesan cheese light for them to coat it.
11. Grease your 13.75" x 10.5" muffin pan and place 3 dough balls in each cup of the pan.

Nutritional info per serving:
Calories: 283 | Fat: 18g | Protein: 17g | Carbs: 6g

Keto bread rolls

These fluffy bread rolls are low carb and gluten free. They can be eaten on their own or used for sandwiches or sliders.
Prep time: 10 minutes | Cooking time: 20 minutes | Serving: 8

Ingredients
- 1 1/3 cups almond flour
- 1 ½ cups shredded mozzarella cheese (part skim)
- 2 oz cream cheese (full fat)
- 1 ½ tbsp baking powder (aluminum free)
- 2 tbsps. coconut flour
- 3 eggs (large)

Instructions:
1. Preheat your oven to 350° F
2. In a clean bowl, put almond flour, coconut flour and baking powder. Mix well and set it aside.
3. Using a microwave-safe bowl, put the cream cheese and mozzarella in it and microwave for 30 seconds. Remove the bowl, stir and microwave again for 30 seconds. This

should go on until the cheese has entirely melted.

4. Using a food processor add the cheese, the eggs and flour mix. Process at high speed for uniformity of the dough. (It is normally sticky.)

5. Knead the dough into a dough ball and separate it into 8 equal pieces. Slightly wet your hands with oil for this step.

6. Roll each piece with your palms to form a ball and place each ball on the baking sheet. (should be 2 inches apart)

7. In a bowl, add the remaining egg and whisk. Brush the egg wash on the rolls.

8. Bake for 20 minutes or until they are golden brown.

Tip: The cheese hardens the rolls thus they should be eaten when hot. Microwave them to make soft once they cool.

Nutritional info per serving:
Calories: 216 | Carbs: 6g | Fat: 16g | Protein: 11g

Keto coconut bread rolls

These easy rolls are made using psyllium husk powder and coconut flour. They are tasty and gluten free.

Prep time: 10 minutes | Cooking time: 30 minutes | Serving: 6

Ingredients
- ½ cup coconut flour
- 4 tbsps. flaxseed (ground)
- 2 tbsps. coconut oil
- 2 tbsps. Powder, psyllium husk
- 1 tbsp baking powder
- 1 tbsp apple cider vinegar
- ¼ cup water, boiled
- ½ tsp salt
- 2 egg whites
- 2 eggs (medium size)

Instructions:
1. Preheat your oven to 350°F.
2. In a mixing bowl, put all your dry ingredients and mix thoroughly. (coconut flour, flaxseed flour, baking powder, psyllium husk powder, salt)
3. Add eggs and the coconut oil. Blend the ingredients till it resembles breadcrumbs. Pour the apple cider vinegar and mix.
4. Add the boiling water in bits. (you don't need to use the entire amount) Stir for it to combine well with the mixture.
5. Line your baking tray with baking paper.
6. Make 6 divisions of the dough and roll them into balls with your hands.
7. Place the dough balls on the baking paper.
8. Bake them for 30 minutes or upon turning to golden brown.

Nutritional info per serving:
Calories: 172 | Carbs: 14g | Fat: 10g | Protein: 10.7g

Low carb bread rolls (without eggs)

These bread rolls are high in protein and fat and will quench your cravings for bread.

Prep time: 15 minutes | Cooking time: 40 minutes | Serving: 6

Ingredients
- ¼ cup coconut flour
- 1 ¼ cup almond flour
- ¼ cup psyllium husk (ground)
- 1 cup hot water
- 1 tbsp olive oil
- 2 tsp apple cider vinegar
- 2 tsps. baking powder
- ½ tsp salt
- 2 tbsps. sesame seeds (optional)

Instructions:
1. Preheat your oven to 375°F.
2. Add all your dry ingredients in a bowl. (Coconut flour, almond flour, psyllium powder, baking powder, salt)
3. Pour the olive oil and apple cider vinegar in the hot water and stir. Thereafter, pour the mix in the bowl and combine thoroughly for a minute. The flour will absorb the water forming the dough. The dough will be soft and sticky. Leave it for 10 minutes for the water mixture to be well absorbed.
4. Separate the dough into 6 equal portions. Form 6 dough balls as a result.
5. Line your baking tray with parchment paper.
6. Place the balls on the baking tray and sprinkle sesame seeds on top. Press the seeds into the dough to prevent falling out.
7. Bake for 40 minutes at 375°F at the lower section of the oven for the first 30

minutes. Switch them to the top section for the remaining period.
8. Remove from the oven and let them cool.
Nutritional info per serving:
Calories: 230 | Carbs: 13.9g | Fat: 18g | Protein: 6.2g

Avocado Mug Bread

This avocado mug bread is naturally green colored, delicious and fluffy.
Prep time: 2 minutes | Cooking time: 2 minutes | Servings: 1
Ingredients:
- ¼ cup Almond Flour
- ½ tsp Baking Powder
- ¼ tsp Salt
- ¼ cup Mashed Avocados
- 1 tbsp Coconut Oil

Instructions:
1. Mix all ingredients in a microwave-safe mug.
2. Microwave for 90 seconds.
3. Cool for 2 minutes.

Nutritional info per serving:
Calories 317 | Carbs 9 g | Fats 30 g | Protein 6 g

Sausage bread

These are soft and light bread that is stuffed with sausage meat. They are indeed crowd pleasers.
Prep time: 10 minutes | Cooking time: 4 hours | Servings: 8
Ingredients:
- 1 ½ teaspoons dry yeast
- 3 cups flour
- 1 teaspoon sugar
- 1 ½ teaspoons salt
- 1 1/3 cups whey
- 1 tablespoon oil
- 1 cup chopped smoked sausage

Instructions:
1. Fold all the ingredients in the order that is recommended specifically for your model.
2. Set the required parameters for baking bread.
3. When ready, remove the delicious hot bread.
4. Wait for it to cool down and enjoy with sausage.

Nutritional info per serving:
Calories 234 | Carbs 4 g | Fats 5.1 g | Protein 7.4 g

Cheese sausage bread

This bread is cheesy, warm and packed with savory flavor. You can serve it with salad or soup.
Prep time: 10 minutes | Cooking time: 4 hours | Servings: 8
Ingredients:
- 1 teaspoon dry yeast
- 3 ½ cups flour
- 1 teaspoon salt
- 1 tablespoon sugar
- 1 ½ tablespoons oil
- 2 tablespoons smoked sausage
- 2 tablespoons grated cheese
- 1 tablespoon chopped garlic
- 1 cup water

Instructions:
1. Cut the sausage into small cubes.
2. Grate the cheese on a grater; chop the garlic.
3. Add the ingredients to the bread machine according to the instructions.
4. Turn on the baking program and let it do the work.

Nutritional info per serving:
Carbs 4 g | Calories 260 | Fats 5.6 g | Protein 7.7 g

Hazelnut honey bread

Yummy and tasty. Give it a try today
Prep time: 10 minutes | Cooking time: 3 hours 10 minutes | Servings: 10
Ingredients:
- ½ cup lukewarm milk
- 2 teaspoons butter, melted and cooled
- 2 teaspoons liquid honey
- 2/3 teaspoons salt
- 1/3 cup cooked wild rice, cooled
- 1/3 cup whole grain flour
- 2/3 teaspoons caraway seeds
- 1 cup almond flour, sifted
- 1 teaspoon active dry yeast
- 1/3 cup hazelnuts, chopped

Instructions:

1. Prepare all of the ingredients for your bread and measuring means (a cup, a spoon, kitchen scales).
2. Carefully measure the ingredients into the pan, except the nuts and seeds.
3. Place all of the ingredients into the bread bucket in the right order, following the manual for your bread machine.
4. Close the cover.
5. Select the program of your bread machine to BASIC and choose the crust color to MEDIUM.
6. Press START.
7. After the signal, add the nuts and seeds into the dough.
8. Wait until the program completes.
9. When done, take the bucket out and let it cool for 5-10 minutes.
10. Shake the loaf from the pan and let cool for 30 minutes on a cooling rack.
11. Slice, serve and enjoy the taste of fragrant homemade bread.

Nutritional info per serving:
Calories 113 | Carbs 5 g | Fats 2.8 g | Protein 3.6 g

Coconut milk bread

Tender, soft and moist sandwich bread flavored with coconut.
Prep time: 10 minutes | Cooking time: 3 hours | Servings: 10

Ingredients:
- 1 whole egg
- ½ cup lukewarm milk
- ½ cup lukewarm coconut milk
- ¼ cup butter, melted and cooled
- 2 tablespoons liquid honey
- 4 cups almond flour, sifted
- 1 tablespoon active dry yeast
- 1 teaspoon salt
- ½ cup coconut chips

Instructions:
1. Prepare all of the ingredients for your bread and measuring means (a cup, a spoon, kitchen scales).
2. Carefully measure the ingredients into the pan, except the coconut chips.
3. Place all of the ingredients into the bread bucket in the right order, following the manual for your bread machine.
4. Close the cover.
5. Select the program of your bread machine to SWEET and choose the crust color to MEDIUM.
6. Press START.
7. After the signal, add the coconut chips into the dough.
8. Wait until the program completes.
9. When done, take the bucket out and let it cool for 5-10 minutes.
10. Shake the loaf from the pan and let cool for 30 minutes on a cooling rack.
11. Slice, serve and enjoy the taste of fragrant homemade bread.

Nutritional info per serving:
Calories 421 | Carbs 6 g | Fats 15.3 g | Protein 9.5 g

Egg bread

This bread is easy to prepare and its delicate and tender.
Prep time: 10 minutes | Cooking time: 3 hours | Servings: 8

Ingredients:
- 4 cups almond flour
- 1 cup milk
- 2 eggs
- 1 teaspoon yeast
- 1 ½ teaspoons salt
- 2 ¼ tablespoons sugar
- 1 ½ tablespoons butter

Instructions:
1. Lay the products in the bread pan according to the instructions for your device. At me in the beginning liquid, therefore we pour warm milk, and we will add salt.
2. Then add the eggs (pre-loosen with a fork) and melted butter, which must be cooled to a warm state.
3. Now add the sifted almond flour.
4. Top the yeast - dry active ones, since they do not require pre-activation with liquid.
5. In the end, mix the yeast with sugar.
6. Select the Basic program (on mine, it is 1 of 12). The time will automatically be set for 3 hours. When the batch begins, this is the most crucial moment. Kneading on this program lasts precisely 10 minutes, from which a ball of all products is produced. Not porridge, not liquid, not a rough dense lump – namely a softball.

7. Ideally, it is formed after the first 4-5 minutes of kneading; then you can help the bread maker. First, scrape off the flour from the walls, which the blade sometimes does not entirely grasp and thus interferes with the dough. Second, you need to look carefully, as different flours from different manufacturers have different degrees of humidity, so it may take a little more - about 2-3 tablespoons. This is when you see that the dough cannot condense and gather in a ball.
8. Very rarely, but sometimes it happens that there is not enough liquid and the dough turns into lumps. If so, add a little more water and thereby help the bread maker knead the dough.
9. After exactly 3 hours, you will hear the signal, but much sooner, your home will be filled with the fantastic aroma of homemade bread. Turn off the appliance, open the lid, and take out the bowl of bread. Handsome!
10. Take out the hot egg bread, and remove the paddle if it does not stay in the bowl, but is at the bottom of the loaf. Cool the loaves on a grate. In general, it is always advised to cool the bread on its side.
11. This bread is quite tall - 12 cm.
12. Only when the loaf completely cools, you can cut the egg bread!
13. Help yourself!

Nutritional info per serving:
Calories 319 | Carbs 3 g | Fats 5.6 g | Protein 9.6 g

Simple keto bread

This keto bread is great for a toast and can be used for sandwiches.
Prep time: 3 minutes | Cooking time: 30 minutes | Servings: 8

Ingredients:
- 3 cups almond flour
- 2 tbsp inulin
- 1 tbsp whole milk
- ½ tsp salt
- 2 tsp active yeast
- 1 ¼ cups warm water
- 1 tbsp olive oil

Instructions:

1. Use a small mixing bowl to combine all dry ingredients, except for the yeast.
2. In the bread machine pan add all wet ingredients.
3. Add all of your dry ingredients, from the small mixing bowl, in the bread machine pan. Top with the yeast.
4. Set the bread machine to the basic bread setting.
5. When the bread is done, remove bread machine pan from the bread machine.
6. Let cool slightly before transferring to a cooling rack.
7. The bread can be stored for up to 5 days on the counter and for up to 3 months in the freezer.

Nutritional info per serving:
Calories 85 | Carbs 4 g | Fats 7 g | Protein 3 g

Multi-grain bread

Delicious and very easy to make.
Prep time: 10 minutes | Cooking time: 6 hours | Servings: 10

Ingredients:
- sugar to taste
- 1 teaspoon salt
- 1 ½ tablespoon olive oil
- 1 ½ teaspoons dry yeast
- 1 ½ tablespoons flower honey
- 1 ½ tablespoons pumpkin seeds
- ½ cup milk
- 1 ½ cups almond flour
- ½ cup barley flour
- ½ cup whole wheat flour
- 1 ½ tablespoon sunflower seeds
- milk to taste
- salt to taste

Instructions:
1. In a small bowl crush the yeast. Rub their hands with 2 tablespoons of wheat flour. Add a pinch of sugar and ½ cup of salted water at room temperature. Cover with a towel and leave for 10 minutes.
2. In the bowl of the bread maker, mix all the remaining flour (pre-sift it), seeds, and nuts. Add the yeast, ¼ cup of warm water, and milk at room temperature. Start mixing the dough. It should be slightly sticky.
3. Add olive oil and honey. Continue to knead. When the dough becomes soft, collect it in one lump, coat with olive oil, and

transfer to a large bowl. Cover it with food film and transfer it to the refrigerator for fermentation for 12 hours.
4. Take the dough out of the refrigerator. Allow it to stand at room temperature for 1 hour. Transfer to the bowl of the bread maker for 1 hour.
5. Lubricate the loaf with milk and sprinkle with salt.
6. Bake in the bread maker according to the instructions. Take the finished bread from the bowl, put it on a grate, and let it cool completely.
Nutritional info per serving:
Calories 179 | Carbs 4 g | Fats 3.7 g | Protein 5.4 g

Toast bread

Simple and tasty snack or breakfast bread.
Prep time: 10 minutes | Cooking time: 3 ½ hours | Servings: 8
Ingredients:
- 1 ½ teaspoons yeast
- 3 cups almond flour
- 2 tablespoons sugar
- 1 teaspoon salt
- 1 ½ tablespoons butter
- 1 cup water

Instructions:
1. Pour water into the bowl; add salt, sugar, soft butter, flour, and yeast.
2. I add dried tomatoes and paprika.
3. Put it on the Basic program.
4. The crust can be light or medium.

Nutritional info per serving:
Calories 203 | Carbs 5 g | Fats 2.7 g | Protein 5.2 g

Walnut bread

A hearty and versatile loaf. Its great for toast for breakfast or thanksgiving.
Prep time: 5 minutes | Cooking time: 4 hours | Servings: 10
Ingredients:
- 4 cups almond flour
- ½ cup water
- ½ cup milk
- 2 eggs
- ½ cup walnuts
- 1 tablespoon vegetable oil
- 1 tablespoon sugar
- 1 teaspoon salt
- 1 teaspoon yeast

Instructions:
1. All products must be room temperature.
2. Pour water, milk, and vegetable oil into the bucket and add in the eggs.
3. Now pour in the sifted almond flour. In the process of kneading bread, you may need a little more or less flour – it depends on its moisture.
4. Pour in salt, sugar, and yeast. If it is hot in the kitchen (especially in summer), pour all three ingredients into the different ends of the bucket so that the dough does not have time for peroxide.
5. Now the first kneading dough begins, which lasts 15 minutes. In the process, we monitor the state of the ball. It should be soft, but at the same time, keep its shape and not spread. If the ball does not want to be collected, add a little flour, since the moisture of this product is different for everyone. If the bucket is clean and all the flour is incorporated into the dough, then everything is done right. If the dough is still lumpy and even crumbles, you need to add a little more liquid.
6. Close the lid and then prepare the nuts. They need to be sorted and lightly fried in a dry frying pan; the pieces of nuts will be crispy. Then let them cool and cut with a knife to the desired size. When the bread maker signals, pour in the nuts and wait until the spatula mixes them into the dough.
7. Remove the bucket and take out the walnut bread. Completely cool it on a grill so that the bottom does not get wet.

Nutritional info per serving:
Calories 257 | Carbs 4 g | Fats 6.7 g | Protein 8.3 g

Bulgur bread

A soft and tender bread with nutty chewiness from bulgur wheat. It slices up beautifully and has a soft crust.
Prep time: 6 minutes | Cooking time: 3 hours | Servings: 8
Ingredients:
- ½ cup bulgur
- 1/3 cup boiling water

- 1 egg
- 1 cup water
- 1 tablespoon butter
- 1 ½ tablespoon milk powder
- 1 tablespoon sugar
- 2 teaspoons salt
- 3 ¼ cup flour
- 1 teaspoon dried yeast

Instructions:
1. Bulgur pour boiling water into a small container and cover with a lid. Leave to stand for 30 minutes.
2. Cut butter into small cubes.
3. Stir the egg with water in a measuring container. The total volume of eggs with water should be 300 ml.
4. Put all the ingredients in the bread maker in the order that is described in the instructions for your bread maker. Bake in the BASIC mode, medium crust.

Nutritional info per serving:
Calories 255 | Carbs 3 g | Fats 3 g | Protein 8.9 g

Italian blue cheese bread

This bread is filled with flavor. Its flavored with butter, cheese and fresh herbs.
Prep time: 10 minutes | Cooking time: 3 hours | Servings: 8

Ingredients:
- 1 teaspoon dry yeast
- 2 ½ cups almond flour
- 1 ½ teaspoon salt
- 1 tablespoon sugar
- 1 tablespoon olive oil
- ½ cup blue cheese
- 1 cup water

Instructions:
1. Mix all the ingredients. Start baking.

Nutritional info per serving:
Carbs 5 g | Fats 4.6 g | Protein 6 g | Calories 194

German bread linz

This bread is great and tasty and perfect to serve with soup. It also freezes well.
Prep time: 8 minutes | Cooking time: 3 ½ hours | Servings: 8

Ingredients
- 2 ¼ cups rye flour
- 2 ¼ cups almond flour

- 1 ¾ cups water + 2 eggs
- 2 teaspoons salt
- 2 tablespoons olive oil (odorless)
- 2 teaspoons dry yeast
- 2 tablespoons honey

Instructions:
2. Crack two eggs into a bowl, and add the rest of the ingredients.
3. Set the program for RYE BREAD or BASIC.
4. Enjoy!

Nutritional info per serving:
Calories 309 | Carbs 3.4 g | Fats 6 g | Protein 10.5 g

Apple bread with horseradish and pistachios

This bread is awesome for fall and makes youe entire houce to smell great.
Prep time: 5 minutes | Cooking time: 3 ½ hours | Servings: 8

Ingredients
- 3 cups almond flour
- 2 eggs
- 3 tablespoons grated horseradish
- ½ cup apple puree/applesauce
- 1 tablespoon sugar
- 4 tablespoons olive oil
- ½ cup chopped pistachios, peeled
- 1 teaspoon dried yeast
- 1 teaspoon salt

Instructions:
1. Lightly beat eggs in a bowl. Pour in enough water to make 280 ml of liquid. Pour into a mold, and add olive oil.
2. Put in the flour, applesauce, horseradish, and half the pistachios. Add salt and sugar from different angles. Make a small groove in the flour and put in the yeast.
3. Bake on the BASIC program. After the final mixing of the dough, moisten the surface of the product with water and sprinkle with the remaining pistachios.
4. Let bread cool.

Nutritional info per serving:
Carbs 2 g | Fats 10.9 g | Protein 7.7 g | Calories 291

Honey bread with cream and coconut milk

This bread is naturally dairy free. You can use frozen fruits for topping and pantry ingredients for the toast.

Prep time: 6 minutes | Cooking time: 3 ½ hours | Servings: 8

Ingredients
- 3 ¾ cups almond flour
- 1 ¾ cups bran meal
- 1 ¼ cups cream
- 1/3 cup coconut milk
- 2 tablespoons honey
- 2 tablespoons vegetable oil
- 2 teaspoons dry yeast
- 2 teaspoons salt

Instructions:
1. Pour in the cream, coconut milk, ½ cup of water, honey, and vegetable oil.
2. Put in the flour and salt. Make a groove in the flour and put in the yeast.
3. Bake on the BASIC program.
4. Cool the bread and serve.

Nutritional info per serving:
Calories 348 | Carbs 4 g | Fats 8.6 g | Protein 8.1 g

Milk almond bread

This is a grain free and delicious bread made with almond flour. It is low in Carbs and high in proteins.

Prep time: 7 minutes | Cooking time: 3 ½ hours | Servings: 8

Ingredients
- 1 ¼ cups milk
- 5 ¼ cups almond flour
- 2 tablespoons butter
- 2 teaspoons dry yeast
- 1 tablespoon sugar
- 2 teaspoons salt

Instructions:
1. Pour the milk into the form and ½ cup of water. Add flour.
2. Put butter, sugar, and salt in different corners of the mold. Make a groove in the flour and put in the yeast.
3. Bake on the Basic program.
4. Cool the bread.

Nutritional info per serving:
Calories 352 | Carbs 5 g | Fats 4.5 g | Protein 10.1 g

Almond bread with a delicate crust

Its dairy free, vegan, low carb and gluten free. This awesome crust is an amazing base of any tart or sweet pie.

Prep time: 8 minutes | Cooking time: 3 ½ hours | Servings: 8

Ingredients
- 1 ¼ cups milk
- 5 ¼ cups almond flour
- 2 tablespoons vegetable oil
- 2 tablespoons sour cream
- 2 teaspoons dried yeast
- 1 tablespoon sugar
- 2 teaspoons salt

Instructions:
1. Pour the milk into the form and ½ cup of water, then add flour.
2. Put butter, sugar, and salt in different corners of the mold. Make a groove in the flour and add the yeast.
3. Bake on the Basic program.
4. After the final mixing of the dough, smear the surface of the product with sour cream.
5. Cool; serve; enjoy.

Nutritional info per serving:
Calories 344 | Carbs 4.5 g | Fats 4.9 g | Protein 8.9 g

Rice bread

This bread has a neutral flavor. It is soft on the inside and crusty on the outside, easy to make and sugar free.

Prep time: 7 minutes | Cooking time: 3 ½ hours | Servings: 8

Ingredients
- 4 ½ cups almond flour
- 1 cup, rice, cooked
- 1 egg
- 2 tablespoons milk powder
- 2 teaspoons dried yeast
- 2 tablespoons butter
- 1 tablespoon sugar
- 2 teaspoons salt

Instructions:
1. Pour 1 ¼ cups of water into the mold; add the egg.
2. Add flour, rice, and milk powder.
3. Put butter, sugar, and salt in different corners of the mold. Make a groove in the flour, and put in the yeast.
4. Bake on the Basic program.

5. When ready, cool the bread.
Nutritional info per serving:
Carbs 5 g | Fats 4.2 g | Protein 9.6 g | Calories 328

Rice bread with soy sauce

This is a yummy bread to eat with soy sauce. Try it today. You will love it
Prep time: 6 minutes | Cooking time: 3 ½ hours | Servings: 8
Ingredients
- 4 ½ cups almond flour
- 1 cup, rice, cooked
- 1 egg
- 2 tablespoons soy sauce
- 2 teaspoons dried yeast
- 2 tablespoons melted butter
- 1 tablespoon brown sugar
- 2 teaspoons salt

Instructions:
1. Pour 1 ¼ cups of water, and soy sauce; add the egg.
2. Put in the flour and rice.
3. Put ghee, sugar, and salt in different corners of the mold. Make a groove in the flour, and put in the yeast.
4. Bake in "normal, medium crust" mode.
5. Bread is ready to eat when cooled.

Nutritional info per serving:
Carbs 3.6 g | Fats 4.2 g | Protein 9.1 g | Calories 321

Cumin bread

This bread is a turn on the white traditional bread recipe with a flavor of cumin.
Prep time: 3 ½ hours | Cooking time: 25 minutes | Servings: 8

Ingredients
- 5 1/3 cups flour
- 1 ½ teaspoons salt
- 1 ½ tablespoons sugar
- 1 tablespoon dry yeast
- 1 ¾ cups water
- 2 tablespoons cumin
- 3 tablespoons sunflower oil

Instructions:
1. Pour warm water into the bucket of the bread maker.
2. Add salt, sugar, and sunflower oil.
3. Sift the almond flour. Pour the sifted flour into the bread maker. Add the yeast.
4. Mix the dough. If the dough turns hard, the bread will turn dense, so add a little water. If the dough turns out too soft, the bread will crumble, so add a little flour. With a wooden spatula, remove the dough from the walls of the bucket.
5. The bread maker can only be opened for the first five minutes and after a signal is sounded to add the herbs. After the signal, add two tablespoons of black cumin.
6. When the program is completed, put the bread on a grate to cool.

Nutritional info per serving:
Carbs 3.1 g | Fats 0.7 g | Protein 9.5 g | Calories 368

Chapter 7: Appetizers & Beverages

Iced Keto Coffee

This Iced keto coffee is a great and tasty treat that keeps you cook on a hot day and is very easy to make.

Prep Time: 5 Minutes | Cooking Time: - | Servings: 1

Ingredients
- 8 oz. cooled strongly brewed coffee.
- 1 scoop collagen peptides.
- 1 tablespoon Brain Octane Oil.
- 2 tablespoons original Nut pods.

Instructions:
1. Add in ingredients like the coffee, collagen peptides and Brain Octane Oil to a medium glass then blend the ingredients together with the aid of a milk frother.
2. Add ice to the mixture then add the nut pods for taste. Stir and enjoy.

Nutritional Info per Serving:
Calories 191 | Fats 16 g | Carbs 0.1 g | Proteins 10.1 g

Jicama Fries

Its paleo, vegan, keto and low carb. For a delicious summer appetizer, serve with guacamole.

Prep time: 45 minutes | Cooking time: 15 minutes | Servings: 2

Ingredients
- 1 jicama, peeled and sliced into thin strips
- 1/2 teaspoon onion powder
- 2 tablespoons avocado oil
- Cayenne pepper, pinch
- 1 teaspoon paprika
- Sea salt, to taste

Instructions:
1. Dry roast the jicama strips in a non-stick frying pan (or you can also grease the pan with a bit of avocado oil)
2. Place the roasted jicama fries into a large bowl and add the onion powder, cayenne pepper, paprika and sea salt.
3. Drizzle over the avocado oil and toss the contents until the flavors are incorporated well.
4. Serve immediately and enjoy!

Nutrition Info per Serving:
Calories 92 | Fats 7 g | Proteins 1 g | Carbs 2 g

Keto Mocha

This smooth and creamy coffee is rich with the chocolate flavor and combines all the benefits of a bulletproof coffee.

Prep Time: 2 minutes | Cooking time: 5 minutes | Servings: 1

Ingredients:
- 2 shots espresso coffee
- 2 teaspoons of MCT oil
- 1 tablespoon of cocoa powder
- 2 teaspoons erythritol
- 2 tablespoons thick cream
- 1/2 cup of keto whipped cream

Instructions:
1. Put the ingredients, MCT oil, cocoa powder and erythritol in a blender.
2. After blending, add a cup of boiling water.
3. Add cream and mix.
4. Serve hot and have fun!

Nutritional Info per serving:
Calories 269 | Fats 29 g | Carbs 1 g | Proteins 1g

Keto Turkish Coffee

This is a great and yummy coffee. You can take it anytime of the day.

Prep time: 5 minutes | Cooking time: - | Servings: 1

Ingredients:
- 1 ½ tablespoons ground coffee beans
- 1 cup hot water
- 1 teaspoon of cardamom
- ½ cup of coconut milk
- Stevia

Instruction:
1. Grind all the coffee beans and cardamom in a coffee grinder.
2. Pour the ground coffee and cardamom into the jar of a coffee maker.
3. Boil water.
4. Pour half of the water in the coffee jar.
5. Wait 30 seconds and mix the water and the ground coffee with a spoon.
6. Pour the rest of the hot water into the container and place the lid on the container.

Nutritional Info per serving:
Calories 69 | Fats 3 g | Carbs 0 g | Proteins 0g

Keto Ice Cream Coffee mix

This is a creamy, rich and low carb coffee ice-cream. It is easy to prepare and sugar free.
Prep Time: 10 minutes | Cooking Time: - | Servings: 1

Ingredients:
- 1 tablespoon of death wish coffee
- 1.5 cup vanilla milk without sugar
- 1 tablespoon of Keto MCT oil
- 1 tablespoon of chia seeds
- 2 tablespoons thick whipped cream
- 1 teaspoon vanilla extract.
- 2 teaspoon Stevia

Instructions:
1. Freeze the coffee in an ice tray.
2. Put all ingredients in a blender and stir until smooth.
3. Pour in a glass. Before serving, wait 5 to 8 minutes for the chia seeds to thicken.

Nutritional Info per serving:
Calories 344 | Fats 32 g | Carbs 7 g | Proteins 4 g

Butter Coffee

Prepare and enjoy this butter coffee anytime.
Prep time: 5 minutes | Cooking time: 5 minutes | Servings: 1

Ingredients
- 1 cup of water
- 2 tablespoons of coffee
- 1 tablespoon of herb-fed butter
- 1 tablespoon of coconut oil

Instructions:
1. Make a cup of coffee your favorite way.
2. Simply simmer the ground coffee in the water for 5 minutes and filter it into a cup. You can also use a French press or a coffee machine!
3. Pour the brewed coffee, butter and coconut oil into the blender.
4. blend for about 10 seconds. You will see that it is immediately light and creamy!
5. Pour the coffee into a cup and enjoy! Add all other ingredients like cinnamon or whipped cream!

Nutritional Info per serving:
Calories 230 | Fats 25 g | Carbs 0 g | Proteins 0 g

Thai Iced Tea

This tea recipe goes best with coconut milk and an organic tea bag
Prep time: 2 minutes | Cooking time: 5 minutes | Servings: 1

Ingredients:
- 1 Thai teabag
- ½ cup of boiling water
- 6-8 ice cubes
- ¼ cup thick cream
- 8 drops of liquid stevia

Instructions:
1. Soak a tea bag in 1/2 cup of boiled water for about 4 to minutes.
2. Take out the tea bag and pour the soaked tea into a glass to serve with 6-8 ice cubes.
3. Pour the thick cream and add liquid stevia. Mix everything and enjoy!

Nutritional Info per serving:
Calories 205 | Fats 21g | Carbs 1g | Proteins 1g

Vanilla Custard

This is a thick, creamy and delicious custard recipe that uses unsweetened almond milk to make it into a low carb dessert.
Prep time: 10 minutes | Cooking time: 10 minutes | Servings: 2

Ingredients
- 8 egg yolks
- 1 cup unsweetened almond milk
- 1 teaspoon vanilla extract
- 10 stevia extract drops (optional)
- 6 tablespoons melted coconut oil or unsalted butter

Instructions:
1. In a large, heatproof bowl, whisk the eggs, and then add the milk, vanilla, and honey.
2. Slowly mix in the melted coconut oil.
3. Now place this bowl over a pan of simmering water.
4. Insert a cooking thermometer into the pudding. Once the thermometer reads 140°F, remove the custard from the water bath.
5. Serve it warm or chilled.

Nutritional Info per serving:
Calories 547 | Fats 54 g | Carbs 4 g | Proteins 12 g

Vanilla Pana Cotta

This dish is a perfectly sweet dessert that satisfies your sweet tooth with its pure and creamy taste.
Prep time: 15 minutes | Cooking time: 5 minutes | Servings: 2
Ingredients:
- 1 teaspoon gelatin powder
- 1 tablespoon water
- 1 cup heavy whipping cream
- ½ tablespoon pure vanilla extract
- 1 tablespoon fresh pomegranate seeds

Instructions:
1. Mix the gelatin powder with the water, and set it aside for 5 minutes.
2. Combine the cream and vanilla extract in a saucepan.
3. Bring the mixture to the boil, then lower the heat and let it simmer.
4. Once the cream begins to thicken, add the gelatin.
5. Stir until the gelatin is dissolved, and pour the cream into serving glasses.
6. Place it in the fridge for two hours, until it is completely cool.
7. Sprinkle the pomegranate seeds on top before serving.

Nutritional Info per serving:
Calories 422 | Fats 43 g | Carbs 4 g | Proteins 4 g

Creamy Cinnamon Coffee

This is a very easy-to-make recipe, with the cozy and warm flavor combo of cinnamon and coffee.
Prep time: 10 minutes | Cooking time: 0 minutes | Servings: 2
Ingredients
- 4 tablespoons instant coffee
- 2 teaspoons ground cinnamon
- 2 cups boiling water
- 1 cup heavy whipping cream
- Stevia liquid extract, optional

Instructions:
1. Mix the coffee and cinnamon together.
2. Add the hot water, and stir.
3. Whip the cream until it is light and fluffy. Add a few drops of stevia if you like your coffee sweet.
4. Serve the coffee in a mug with the whipping cream on top.

Nutritional Info per serving:
Calories 136 | Fats 14 g | Carbs 2 g | Protein 1 g

Chia Seed Pudding

A sweet, low carb and luxurious treat to enjoy.
Prep time: 5 minutes | Cooking time: 0 minutes | Servings: 2
Ingredients
- 1 ½ cup coconut milk
- 4 tablespoons Chia seeds
- 1 teaspoon pure vanilla extract
- 10 drops stevia extract

Instructions:
1. Combine all the ingredients in a large jar.
2. Cover the jar and place it in the refrigerator to chill.
3. Once the pudding thickens and the chia seeds have gelled, serve the pudding with whipped cream.

Nutritional Info per Serving
Calories 186 | Fats 13 g | Carbs 16 g | Protein 7 g

Tasty Chicken Egg Rolls

These are just what you need! It's the best keto party appetizer!
Prep time: 2 hours and 10 minutes | Cooking time: 15 minutes | Servings: 12
Ingredients:
- 4 ounces blue cheese
- 2 cups chicken, cooked and finely chopped
- Salt and black pepper to the taste
- 2 green onions, chopped
- 2 celery stalks, finely chopped
- ½ cup tomato sauce
- ½ teaspoon erythritol
- 12 egg roll wrappers
- Vegetable oil

Instructions:
1. In a bowl, mix chicken meat with blue cheese, salt, pepper, green onions, celery, tomato sauce and sweetener, stir well and keep in the fridge for 2 hours.
2. Place egg wrappers on a working surface, divide chicken mix on them, roll and seal edges.
3. Heat up a pan with vegetable oil over medium high heat, add egg rolls, cook until they are golden, flip and cook on the other side as well.
4. Arrange on a platter and serve them.

Nutritional Info per serving:
Calories 220 | Fats 7 g | Carbs 6 g | Protein 10 g

Avocado Gazpacho

This is a cool summer soup that is made with Greek yogurt, sweet onions and cucumbers.
Prep time: 15 minutes | Servings: 2 |
Ingredients:
- 2 avocados, peeled, pitted and chopped
- 3 tablespoons fresh cilantro leaves
- 1½ cups homemade vegetable broth
- 1 tablespoon fresh lemon juice
- ½ teaspoon ground cumin
- 1/8 teaspoon cayenne pepper
- Salt, as required

Instructions:
1. Add all the ingredients in a high-speed blender and pulse until smooth.
2. Transfer the gazpacho into a large bowl.
3. Cover the bowl and refrigerate to chill completely before serving.

Nutritional Info per serving:
Calories 235 | Fats 20.7 g | Carbs 9.4 g | Proteins 5.6 g

Spinach Chips

It's an exceptional keto appetizer recipe!
Prep time: 5 minutes | Cooking time: 15 minutes | Servings: 6
Ingredients:
- 1 tablespoon olive oil
- 1-pound baby spinach
- ½ teaspoon curry powder
- A pinch of salt and black pepper
- ½ teaspoon cumin, ground

Instructions:
1. In a bowl, mix the spinach leaves with the oil and the other ingredients and toss gently.
2. Spread the basil leaves well on a baking sheet lined with parchment paper, and cook in the oven at 420 degrees F for 15 minutes.
3. Cool down and serve as a snack.

Nutritional Info per serving:
Calories 30 | Fats 3 g | Carbs 0.5 g | Protein 1 g

Parsley Dip

This is flavored and delicious!
Prep time: 5 minutes | Cooking time: 0 minutes | Servings: 6
Ingredients:
- 1 cup parsley
- 2 tablespoons pine nuts, toasted
- 2 tablespoons olive oil
- 3 ounces heavy cream
- ¼ teaspoon garlic powder
- A pinch of salt and black pepper
- 1 chili pepper, chopped

Instructions:
1. In a blender, combine the parsley with the pine nuts and the other ingredients, pulse well, divide into small bowls and serve as a dip.

Nutritional Info per serving:
Calories 130 | Fats 3.8 g | Carbs 2.2 g | Protein 5 g

Kale Muffins

This is a great keto appetizer!
Prep time: 10 minutes | Cooking time: 30 minutes | Servings: 6
Ingredients:
- 1 cup almond flour
- Salt and black pepper to the taste
- 2 eggs
- 2 tablespoons coconut oil, melted
- 1 teaspoon baking powder
- 1 cup heavy cream
- 1 cup kale, chopped
- A pinch of salt and black pepper

Instructions:
1. In a bowl, the flour with the eggs and the other ingredients, whisk well and divide into a muffin tray.
2. Introduce in the oven at 350 degrees F, bake for 30 minutes and serve cold as a snack or appetizer.

Nutritional info per serving:
Calories 247 | Fats 22.3 g | Carbs 6.2 g | Protein 6.6 g

Cream Cheese Spread

You will love this great spread!
Prep time: 10 minutes | Cooking time: 25 minutes | Servings: 4
Ingredients:
- 6 ounces cream cheese, soft
- ¼ cup parmesan, grated
- A pinch of salt and black pepper
- 1 tablespoon basil, chopped
- 1 tablespoon chives, chopped
- 1 teaspoon sweet paprika

Instructions:
1. In a bowl, combine the cream cheese with the parmesan and the other ingredients, whisk well and divide into 4 ramekins.

2. Introduce in the oven at 360 degrees F, bake for 25 minutes and serve cold.
Nutritional Info per serving:
Calories 200 | Fats 5.4 g | Carbs 5.4 g | Proteins: 5.5 g

Beef Muffins

Everyone appreciates a great treat and this is it
Prep time: 10 minutes | Cooking time: 30 minutes | Servings: 6
Ingredients:
- ½ cup coconut flour
- 1-pound beef, ground and browned
- 2 eggs, whisked
- A pinch of salt and black pepper
- 2 spring onions, chopped
- Cooking spray
- ¼ teaspoon baking powder
- ¼ cup coconut milk

Instructions:
1. In a bowl, combine the meat with the flour and the other ingredients except the cooking spray and stir well.
2. Grease a muffin tray with the cooking spray, divide the beef mix in each muffin mold, introduce in the oven at 360 degrees F and bake for 30 minutes.
3. Serve as an appetizer.
Nutritional Info per serving:
Calories 227 | Fats 9.7 g | Carbs 7.8 g | Proteins 26.4 g

Herbs Spread

Try this herbed appetizer today!
Prep time: 10 minutes | Cooking time: 0 minutes | Servings: 8
Ingredients:
- 1 cup cream cheese, soft
- ½ cup cheddar cheese, grated
- 2 tablespoons olive oil
- 2 tablespoons oregano, chopped
- 1 tablespoon chives, chopped
- 1 tablespoon rosemary, chopped
- 1 tablespoon parsley, chopped
- ¼ teaspoon garlic powder
- A pinch of salt and black pepper
- ¼ teaspoon sweet paprika

Instructions:
1. In a blender, combine the cream cheese with the cheddar and the other ingredients, pulse well, divide into small bowls and serve.
Nutritional Info per serving:
Calories 150 | Fats 6.3 g | Carbs 5.1 g | Protein 2 g

Thyme Leek Snack Bowls

This is a simple, yet very tasty keto appetizer
Prep time: 10 minutes | Cooking time: 30 minutes | Servings: 8
Ingredients:
- 2 tablespoons olive oil
- 3 leeks, sliced
- A pinch of salt and black pepper
- 2 teaspoons garlic, minced
- 1 tablespoon thyme, chopped
- 2 tablespoons parmesan, grated

Instructions:
1. In a bowl, combine the leek slices with the oil and the other ingredients except the parmesan and toss.
2. Spread the leeks on a baking sheet lined with parchment paper, sprinkle the cheese on top, introduce in the oven at 420 degrees F and bake for 30 minutes.
3. Divide into bowls and serve as a snack.
Nutritional Info per serving:
Calories 163 | Fats 13 g | Proteins 3 g | Carbs 5.3 g

Cilantro and Leeks Dip

This is not a guacamole! It's much better
Prep time: 10 minutes | Cooking time: 0 minutes | Servings: 4
Ingredients:
- ¼ cup cilantro, chopped
- 2 leeks, sliced
- Juice of 1 lime
- A pinch of salt and black pepper
- ½ cup coconut oil, melted
- ½ cup cream cheese, soft

Instructions:
1. In a blender, combine the leeks with the cilantro and the other ingredients, pulse well, divide into small cups and serve as a party dip.!
Nutritional Info per serving:
Calories 150 | Fats 14 g | Proteins 2 g | Carbs 4 g

Shrimp Bowls

You've got to love this!
Prep time: 10 minutes | Cooking time: 10 minutes | Servings: 6
Ingredients:
- 2 tablespoons olive oil

- 1-pound shrimp, peeled and deveined
- 1 tablespoons mint, chopped
- A pinch of salt and black pepper
- 1 teaspoon smoked paprika
- 1 cup baby spinach
- 1 avocado, peeled, pitted and cubed
- 1 tablespoon lime juice

Instructions:
1. Spread the shrimp on a baking sheet lined with parchment paper, season with salt, pepper and the paprika, drizzle half of the oil, and bake at 400 degrees F for 10 minutes.
2. Transfer the shrimp to a bowl, add the rest of the ingredients, toss, divide into smaller bowls and serve as an appetizer.

Nutritional Info per serving:
Calories 245 | Fats 12 g | Carbs 1 g | Protein 14 g

Cheddar Cauliflower Bites

This snack will really make you feel full for a couple of hours!
Prep time: 10 minutes | Cooking time: 25 minutes | Servings: 8

Ingredients:
- 1-pound cauliflower florets
- 1 teaspoon sweet paprika
- A pinch of salt and black pepper
- 2 eggs, whisked
- 1 cup coconut flour
- Cooking spray
- 1 cup cheddar cheese, grated

Instructions:
1. In a bowl, mix the flour with salt, pepper, the cheese and the paprika and stir.
2. Put the eggs in a separate bowl.
3. Dredge the cauliflower florets in the eggs and then in the cheese mix, arrange them on a baking sheet lined with parchment paper and bake at 380 degrees F for 25 minutes.
4. Serve.

Nutritional Info per serving:
Calories 163 | Fats 12 g | Carbs 2 g | Proteins 7 g

Turmeric Dip

This is so delicious and simple to make!
Prep time: 10 minutes | Cooking time: 0 minutes | Servings: 4

Ingredients:
- 2 tablespoons olive oil
- 1 cup cream cheese, soft
- 1 teaspoon turmeric powder
- 1 tablespoon cilantro, chopped
- Salt and black pepper to the taste
- A pinch of cayenne pepper

Instructions:
1. In a blender, combine the cream cheese with the turmeric and the other ingredients, pulse well, divide into small cups and serve.

Nutritional Info per serving:
Calories 345 | Fats 33 g | Carbs 5 g | Proteins 16 g

Tomato Dip

Try this today! You'll love it
Prep time: 10 minutes | Cooking time: 15 minutes | Servings: 4

Ingredients:
- 1 cup cream cheese, soft
- ¼ cup tomato passata
- 1 tablespoon basil, chopped
- ½ teaspoon sweet paprika
- Salt and black pepper to the taste

Instructions:
1. In a bowl, combine the cream cheese with the passata and the other ingredients, whisk well, divide into 4 ramekins, introduce in the oven at 370 degrees F and bake for 15 minutes.
2. Serve cold.

Nutritional Info per serving:
Calories 140 | Fats 4 g | Carbs 6 g | Proteins 4 g

Chapter 8: Desserts

Cheesecake Bites

This is a delicious dessert loved by everyone. Its nestled by a rich and creamy cheesecake filling.
Prep time: 1 hour 10 minutes | Servings: 15
Ingredients:
- ½ cup allulose
- 4 oz. butter, softened
- ½ tsp. vanilla extract, sugar-free
- 8 oz. cream cheese, softened

Instructions:
1. Use a mini cupcake pan and line with baking cups. Set to the side.
2. In a stand mixer on high, cream the sweetener and butter for approximately 3 minutes.
3. Blend the vanilla extract and cream cheese until incorporated.
4. Spoon the mixture into the baking cups and freeze for 1 hour until firm.
5. No need to wait for them to defrost. Serve and enjoy!

Nutritional Info Per Serving:
Calories 107 | Fat 11.4g | Carbs 0.4g | Protein 1.2g

Chocolate Chip Balls

Easy to make and very sweet.
Prep time: 1 hour 10 minutes | Servings: 16
Ingredients:
- 4 tbsp. cocoa powder, unsweetened
- ½ cup allulose
- 4oz. butter, unsalted and softened
- 8oz. cream cheese, softened
- ¼ cup chocolate chips, unsweetened
- 4 tbsp. cup water

Instructions:
1. Using baking paper or a non-stick mat, cover a cooking sheet and set to the side.
2. In a food blender set on medium, cream the water and cocoa powder for 3 minutes.
3. Combine the allulose, cream cheese, and butter. Turn the setting for the food processor to high and whisk for 4 additional minutes.
4. Use a rubber scraper to blend in the unsweetened chocolate chips.
5. Measure out the batter with a 1-inch cookie scoop and drop on the prepared cookie sheet.
6. The balls need to be frozen for 1 hour.
7. Remove from the freezer 10 minutes before serving.

Nutritional Info Per Serving:
Calories 117 | Fat 11.7g | Carbs 2.7g | Protein 1.6g

Coconut Bars

They are tastier and crispier. Make them today
Prep time: 45 minutes | Servings: 2
Ingredients:
- 1 large scoop protein powder, vanilla flavored
- 4 oz. dark chocolate chips, unsweetened
- 1 cup coconut, flaked
- ¾ cup coconut oil, melted
- 1½ cups macadamia nuts, raw

Instructions:
1. Using an 8-inch pan, cover with baking paper or a non-stick mat.
2. In a food blender set to high, blend the macadamia nuts and coconut oil until evenly mixed.
3. Combine the protein powder, chocolate chips, and coconut until mixed thoroughly.
4. Transfer the batter to the prepped pan and freeze for half an hour.
5. After it's set, slice into 14 individual bars.
6. Thaw for 10 minutes before serving.

Nutritional Info Per Serving:
Calories 1417 | Fat 147.8g | Carbs 28.7g| Protein 16.9g

Frozen Yogurt

With just few ingredients, enjoy the sweetness of this frozen yogurt.
Prep time: 35 minutes | Servings: 8
Ingredients:
- 3 cups plain yogurt, full fat and chilled
- 1 tbsp. MCT oil
- 2 tsp. vanilla extract, sugar-free
- 1 tbsp. lemon juice

- 4 tbsp. monk fruit sweetener

Instructions:
1. In a food blender set on medium, blend the lemon juice, MCT oil, and sweetener for 2 minutes until incorporated.
2. Add the yogurt and vanilla extract and stir in with a rubber scraper.
3. Place the bowl in the freezer for half an hour.
4. Serve and enjoy.

Nutritional Info Per Serving:
Calories 81 | Fat 2.9g | Carbs 7.1g | Protein 5.3g

Key Lime Pie

This treat makes an indulgent and refreshing end to a meal. It has a cream. Lime and buttery biscuit base.

Prep time: 4 hours 15 minutes | Servings: 6

Ingredients:
- 3 tsp. allulose
- ½ cup pecans, raw and finely chopped
- 3 tsp. butter, unsalted
- ½ cup heavy whipping cream
- 3 tbsp. lime juice
- ¼ cup + 2 tbsp. stevia
- 4 oz. cream cheese, softened
- ¼ tsp. salt
- 6 lime slices

Instructions:
1. Set out a cupcake pan and line with baker or non-stick cups.
2. In a food blender set on medium, whip the cream cheese, lime juice, and ¼ cup stevia until creamed.
3. In a regular sized dish, combine and mix the remaining 2 tablespoons of stevia and heavy whipping cream for 3 minutes.
4. Combine the whipped cream and cream cheese mixture using a rubber scraper.
5. Heat a small saucepan and melt the butter, allulose, and pecans for 6 minutes. Stir in the salt and remove from heat.
6. Transfer the lime mixture to the cupcake cups and top with pecans.
7. Freeze for 4 hours to set. Remove the paper liner before serving.

Nutritional Info Per Serving:
Calories 140 | Fat 12.5g | Carbs 8.2g | Protein 2.2g

Raspberry Ice Cream

This ice-cream is so easy to make and so yummy.

Prep time: 10 minutes | Servings: 5

Ingredients:
- 2 cups raspberries, frozen
- 1/3 cup stevia, confectioner
- 1 cup heavy whipping cream

Instructions:
1. Using a food processor on high, whisk the heavy whipping cream for 4 minutes.
2. Combine the raspberries and sweetener and puree for 2 additional minutes.
3. Taste test to ensure the sweetness is to your preference. Add 1 – 2 tablespoons of stevia, if required and stir again.
4. Spoon into serving dishes and enjoy!

Nutritional Info Per Serving:
Calories 108 | Fat 9.2g | Carbs 6.5g | Protein 1.1g

Yogurt Popsicles

These healthy and simple treats will keep you feeling cool the entire summer. Try them today.

Prep time: 1 hour 5 minutes | Servings: 6

Ingredients:
- 1 tsp. vanilla extract, sugar-free
- 1 cup Greek yogurt
- 8 oz. strawberries, diced
- ½ cup heavy whipping cream

Instructions:
1. In a food processor set on high, whip the yogurt until fluffy.
2. Blend the strawberries, vanilla extract and heavy whipping cream until smooth.
3. Transfer to popsicle molds and freeze for 1 hour.

Nutritional Info Per Serving:
Calories 96 | Fat 4.6g | Carbs 10.3g | Protein 4.1g

Vanilla Berry Mug Cake

This cake is just less than net carb of 5 g. It is easy and quick to make.

Prep time: 3 minutes | Cooking Time: 1 minutes | Servings: 1

Ingredients:
- 6 frozen raspberries
- 2 tbsp coconut flour

- 1/4 tsp baking powder
- 1 tbsp butter, melted
- 1 egg medium
- 1 tbsp granulated sweetener
- 2 tbsp cream cheese
- 1 tsp vanilla extract

Instructions:
1. Microwave the cream cheese and butter together in a mug on high for 20 seconds.
2. Add the baking powder, coconut flour, vanilla extract and granulated sweetener to the butter and cream cheese mixture. Mix until all the ingredients are combined.
3. Add the egg to the mixture and keep mixing until fully combined and smooth batter is prepared.
4. Add the frozen raspberries and press them gently from the top.
5. Place in the microwave and keep on high for 2 minutes.
6. Enjoy the amazing vanilla berry mug cake.

Nutritional Info Per Serving:
Calories 330 | Fat 14.5g | Carbs 38.3g | Protein 11.5g

Pumpkin Spice Mug Cake

This recipe is an easy and quick way to get you the fix of the pumpkin without you tearing the entire kitchen.
Prep time: 4 minutes | Cooking Time: 1 minute | Servings: 1

Ingredients:
- 1 egg
- 2 tbsp almond meal
- 2 tsp granulated erythritol
- 2 tbsp butter
- 2 tsp pumpkin spice
- 1 tbsp coconut flour
- 1 tbsp heavy cream
- ¼ tsp baking powder

Instructions:
1. Put butter in a microwave bowl and microwave it for half a minute or until melted.
2. Remove the bowl from the microwave once butter is melted.
3. Add coconut flour, baking powder, almond meal and pumpkin spice to the melted butter and mix until well combined.
4. Add egg, butter, heavy cream and erythritol to the mixture and keep mixing until fully combined.
5. Place the bowl again in the microwave to cook the mixture on high for a minute.
6. Remove from the microwave once cooked.
7. Transfer to the serving mug and enjoy the delicious, moist and fluffy pumpkin spice mug cake with heavy cream at the top.

Nutritional Info Per Serving:
Calories 460 | Fat 41.3g | Carbs 22.3g | Protein 10.8g

Lemon Coconut Cake

The lemon coconut cake is made of homemade lemon curd, cream cheese frosting and toasted coconut. Its tender and moist.
Prep time: 10 minutes | Cooking Time: 1 hour 50 minutes | Servings: 12

Ingredients:
For the cake:
- 1 cup Erythritol
- 2 ½ tsp. baking powder, gluten-free
- ½ cup Almond Flour Sukrin
- 1 cup butter, unsalted and room temperature
- 2 ½ cups almond flour, finely milled
- 2 cups coconut, unsweetened and flaked
- ½ cup grated lemon
- ½ cup heavy whipping cream
- 2 tsp. ground ginger
- 1 cup pecans, raw and roughly chopped
- 5 large eggs
- ½ tsp. ground nutmeg
- 2 tbsp. cinnamon powder
- ½ tsp. salt

For the frosting:
- ¾ cup heavy whipping cream
- 1 ¼ cup swerve
- ¾ cup unsalted butter, softened
- 12 oz. cream cheese, full fat

For the topping:
- 1 cup pecans, raw and roughly chopped

Instructions:
Cake:

1. Set your stove to the temperature of 350° Fahrenheit. Use cooking spray or heavily butter the sides and base of two 9-inch cake pans. Cover them with baking paper.
2. In a regular dish, blend the sweetener and butter until mixed well. Add 1 egg and beat into the mixture and repeat until all eggs are combined.
3. Stir the heavy whipping cream, brown sugar and carrots into the batter until thoroughly incorporated.
4. In a big dish, whisk the almond flour remove the lumps if present.
5. Then add the cinnamon powder, ground nutmeg, baking powder, and ground ginger.
6. Slowly combine the flour to the cake batter. Incorporate the coconut and pecans until mixed together.
7. Evenly distribute the batter in the prepared cake pans and heat in the stove for 35 minutes. Use a toothpick in the middle of the cake to make sure it is baked properly.
8. Remove to the counter and let it rest for 10 minutes. Unlock the pan and set the cake to the side until ready to frost.

Frosting:
1. Using a food processor on high, whisk the butter, sweetener and cream cheese for 3 minutes. Scrape the dish with a rubber scraper as necessary and continue to blend until fully incorporated.
2. Pour the heavy whipping cream into the frosting and beat for an additional 2 minutes until airy.
3. Move the first layer on a cake platter and apply the frosting to the top, keeping an even layer. Put the second cake above and apply frosting to the top.
4. Then frost the edges of the layers of cake keeping the frosting as even as possible.
5. Dust the top with the chopped pecans, cut into slices and serve.

Nutritional Info Per Serving:
Calories 816 | Fat 84.2g | Carbs 19.4g | Protein 11g

No Bake Coconut Bars

These bars have no refined sugar. It can be topped with crunchy dark chocolate.
Prep time: 10 minutes | Cooking Time: 90 minutes | Servings: 5

Ingredients:
- 4 tbsp coconut cream
- 10 tbsp shredded coconut
- 4 tbsp erythritol
- 2.10 oz chocolate chips

Instructions:
1. Take a small mixing bowl, add coconut cream, shredded coconut, erythritol, keep mixing until you get a crumbly and thick mixture.
2. Take a silicone mold in rectangular shape and transfer the prepared mixture into that, leaving a 0.2-inch space for the melted chocolate.
3. Place in the fridge to chill for half an hour.
4. Melt the chocolate with the help of double boiler and pour it at the top of chilled coconut filling in the silicone mold.
5. Place in the fridge to chill for another half hour.
6. Line a baking tray with parchment paper, get the bars released from the mold and transfer them into the baking tray.
7. Drop some melted chocolate at the top of each bar and place in the fridge once gain for half an hour.
8. Pull out of the fridge once ready and enjoy the delicious coconut bars.

Nutritional Info Per Serving:
Calories 127 | Fat 9.7g | Carbs 18.9g | Protein 1.5g

Peanut Butter Bars

These butter peanuts bars taste just like butter cups.
Prep time: 15 minutes | Cooking Time: 2 hours, 30 minutes | Servings: 6

Ingredients:
Peanut Butter Base:
- 5 tbsp almond flour
- 4 tbsp granulated erythritol
- ½ cup natural peanut butter
- 1 tsp vanilla extract
- 4 tbsp butter, melted

Topping:
- 2.50 oz sugar-free chocolate
- ¼ cup Chopped peanuts

Instructions:

1. Take a large mixing bowl, add almond flour, erythritol, butter, peanut butter, vanilla extract and mix until smooth.
2. Transfer the mixture to the silicone mold, leaving 0.2-inch space for melted chocolate.
3. Place in the freezer to chill for 30 minutes.
4. Melt the chocolate with the help of double boiler and pour a part of it at the top of peanut butter filling in the silicone mold.
5. Place in the freezer again for 2 hours or until the bars get hard.
6. Remove from the freezer once hard, get the bars released from the silicone mold and transfer them to the baking rack lined with parchment paper.
7. Heat the remaining melted chocolate and pour it over the bars, making sure that each bar is covered completely.
8. Spread chopped peanuts at the top and place in the freezer once again for 1 hour or until hard.
9. Remove from the freezer once ready and enjoy the delicious peanut butter bars.

Nutritional Info Per Serving:
Calories 329 | Fat 27.8g | Carbs 21.6g | Protein 9.2g

Coconut Chocolate Bars

This is a crowd pleasig dessert and easy to make. The combinations of flavor cant be much better than coconut anc chocolate.
Prep time: 10 minutes | Cooking Time: 25 minutes | Servings: 16

Ingredients:
- 1 large egg
- 2 ounces unsweetened desiccated coconut
- 4 ounces unsalted butter, melted
- 3 ounces almond flour
- 1 teaspoon vanilla extract
- 3 ounces maple syrup
- 1 tbsp unsweetened shredded coconut
- 1/2 tsp baking powder
- 2 tbsp unsweetened cocoa powder

Frosting:
- 1 tbsp unsalted butter, melted
- 2 tbsp hot water
- 2 tbsp unsweetened cocoa powder

Instructions:
1. Preheat oven to 340°F and get a 7x11 baking tin ready by lining with parchment paper.
2. Take a mixing bowl, add cocoa powder, baking powder, desiccated coconut and mix all the ingredients until combined.
3. Add vanilla extract, egg and melted butter to the mixture and keep mixing until fully combined.
4. Transfer the mixture to the baking tin and make it even from the top using a spatula.
5. Place in the oven and bake for 25 minutes or until you feel springing back upon touching.
6. To prepare the frosting, add cocoa powder and surkin melis in a mixing bowl through a sifter.
7. Add melted butter and hot water to the mixture and keep stirring until it is ready to be spread.
8. Remove from the oven when properly baked, spread the frosting at the top and allow to cool.
9. Sprinkle the shredded coconut, cut into bars and enjoy.

Nutritional Info Per Serving:
Calories 121 | Fat 10.6g | Carbs 6g | Protein 1.7g

Chocolate Fudge Bars

If you want to have a healthy dessert which requires no baking, melts your mouth and is quick. The chocolate fudge bars are indeed the recipe you can try today.
Prep time: 7 minutes | Cooking Time: 15 minutes | Servings: 16

Ingredients:
- 8 oz. chocolate chips, unsweetened
- ½ cup peanut butter

Instructions:
1. Cover an 8 square inch pan with baking lining and set to the side.
2. Heat a saucepan to melt the chocolate chips until liquefied. Then blend in the peanut butter until the batter is smooth.
3. Distribute to the prepped pan and level out with a rubber scraper
4. Put the fudge into the freezer for 10 minutes to firm.
5. Slice and enjoy!

Nutritional Info Per Serving:

Calories 123 | Fat 8.3g | Carbs 10g | Protein 3.1g

Granola Bars

A soft, simple and chewy granora bars are so delicous and can be adapted basing on your favourite nuts, dried fruits or chocolate.
Prep time: 8 minutes | Cooking Time: 30 minutes | Servings: 8 Bars

Ingredients:
For the granola:
- 1/3 cup monk fruit sweetener
- 2 tsp. vanilla extract, sugar-free
- ¼ cup coconut oil
- ½ cup almonds, sliced
- ¼ cup coconut, unsweetened and shredded
- 1/3 cup flaxseed meal
- ½ cup almond butter, smooth
- 1/3 cup pumpkin seeds, shelled
- 1 tbsp. chia seeds
- ½ tsp. ground cinnamon

For the drizzle:
- 1 tsp. coconut oil
- 3 tbsp. dark chocolate chips, sugar-free

For the topping:
- 1 tbsp. almonds, sliced

Instructions:
1. Using a regular loaf pan, layer with baking paper and set to the side.
2. Heat a pot to liquefy the sweetener, coconut oil, almond butter, and vanilla extract.
3. In a big dish, combine the almonds and coconut with a rubber scraper. Then add the flaxseed meal, pumpkin seeds, chia seeds, and cinnamon to fully incorporate.
4. Transfer the granola to the prepared pan and press down the mixture by hand to make uniform.
5. Freeze the granola for 20 minutes to harden.
6. In a saucepan, dissolve the chocolate chips and coconut oil together.
7. When set, remove and move the granola onto a serving plate.
8. Dust the almonds on the top and drizzle the chocolate over the almonds. Freeze for 3 additional minutes.
9. Cut into 8 individual bars and enjoy!

Nutritional Info Per Serving:
Calories 491 | Fat 47.3g | Carbs 15.2g | Protein 5.8g

Lemon Bars

Lemon bars are extra creamy and so thick. Perfect for baby showers, bake sales, picnics, bridal showers and more.
Prep time: 8 minutes | Cooking Time: 1 hour | Servings: 8

Ingredients:
- 1 cup allulose
- 3 large eggs
- ¼ tsp. salt
- 1 ¾ cups almond flour
- 3 medium lemons
- ½ cup butter, melted

Instructions:
1. Set your stove to the temperature of 350° Fahrenheit. Cover an 8-inch cake pan with baking paper and set to the side.
2. In a big dish, blend 1 cup of the almond flour and butter until fully incorporated. Add the allulose (1/4 cup) and salt (1/8 teaspoon) and combine completely.
3. Push the batter squarely into the prepped pan and heat for 20 minutes. Remove and set on a heat resistant surface while mixing the filling.
4. Zest 1 lemon in a dish and add the juice from all 3 lemons. Add the remaining 3/4 cup almond flour and mix well.
5. Add 1 egg and cream into the mixture, repeating for all the eggs.
6. Finally, add the allulose (3/4 cup) and salt (1/8 teaspoon) and incorporate thoroughly.
7. Transfer the filling to the cooled baking pan and heat in the stove for 25 more minutes.
8. Remove and dust the top with allulose and garnish with a slice of lemon, if preferred.

Nutritional Info Per Serving:
Calories 381 | Fat 24.9g | Carbs 33.8g | Protein 7.7g

Chocolate Cake

You cant find a chocolate cake recipe better than this. Its goodness is so amazing and its so yummy.

Prep time: 10 minutes | Cooking Time: 10 hours 5 minutes | Servings: 12

Ingredients:
For the filling:
- 2 ¾ cup almond flour
- 1 ½ cups sweetener, granulated
- 2 tsp. baking powder, gluten-free
- ½ cup butter, melted
- 4 oz. dark chocolate, stevia sweetened
- ½ cup cocoa powder, unsweetened
- 6 large eggs
- 1 avocado, pureed
- 2 tsp. vanilla extract, sugar-free
- 1 tsp. salt

For the icing:
- ½ cup butter
- liquid stevia, to taste
- ½ cup cocoa powder, unsweetened
- 1/8 tsp. salt

Instructions:
Cake:
1. Set your stove to the temperature of 350° Fahrenheit. Use cooking spray or heavily butter an 8-inch cake pan or cover with parchment lining.
2. In a regular dish, combine the eggs, avocado, baking powder, and vanilla extract until mixed well.
3. Add the almond flour, sweetener, dark chocolate and butter until incorporated. Then add the salt and cacao powder until smooth.
4. Distribute the cake batter into the prepped pan and heat in the stove for 45 minutes. Using a wooden stick, press it into the middle of the cake to make sure it is baked properly.
5. Transfer to the counter and remove from the pan. Set to the side.

Frosting:
1. Heat a saucepan to liquefy the butter completely.
2. Combine the cacao powder, salt, and liquid stevia and mix until smooth.
3. Let the icing completely cool before frosting the cake.
4. Remember to frost the middle first. Then to complete the frosting, down the sides.

Nutritional Info Per Serving:

Calories 515 | Fat 36.7g | Carbs 41.2g | Protein 10.8g

Cinnamon & Nutmeg Cake

This cake is very easy to make. Cinnamon and nutmeg produce a very good flavor.

Prep time: 1 hour 15 minutes | Cooking Time: 40 minutes | Servings: 14

Ingredients:
For the cake:
- 1 ½ cups almond flour
- 5 oz. butter, unsalted and softened
- 1 tsp. ground cinnamon
- ¾ cup sweetener, granulated
- 1 tsp. baking powder, gluten-free
- 2 tbsp. coconut flour
- ½ tsp. ground ginger
- 5 oz. cream cheese, softened
- ¼ sp. ground cloves
- ½ tsp. ground nutmeg
- 5 large eggs
- 1/8 tsp. salt

For the icing:
- 2/3 cup Natvia icing mix
- 4 oz. butter, unsalted and softened
- 2 tbsp. heavy whipping cream
- 4 oz. cream cheese, softened
- 1 tsp. ground cinnamon

Instructions:
Cake:
1. Set the temperature of the stove to 350° Fahrenheit. Use butter to liberally grease an 8-inch cake pan and place baking paper to cover the base of the cake pan.
2. In a big dish, blend the cream cheese and baking powder using an electrical beater.
3. Add the butter and sweetener until combined. Then sprinkle the cinnamon, cloves, nutmeg, and salt into the mixture.
4. Combine the almond flour, coconut flour, and eggs making sure there are no lumps present. Use a scraper on the dish and thoroughly mix.
5. Distribute the cake batter in the prepared pan and heat in the stove for 30 – 40 minutes. Ensure it is baked all the way through by poking a toothpick into the middle.
6. Remove the pan and place on the cake platter. Set to the side.

Frosting:

1. In a regular dish, blend cream cheese until the mixture is creamy.
2. Combine the butter and mix thoroughly.
3. Add the Natvia icing mix one spoonful at a time to ensure it gets completely mixed. Then combine the heavy whipping cream and cinnamon, continuing to stir the frosting until smooth.
4. Frost the middle first and then complete the frosting process after the cake has completely cooled.

Nutritional Info Per Serving:
Calories 341 | Fat 31.2g | Carbs 9.8g | Protein 6.4g

Coffee Cake

This is a perfect cake to have on Sunday mornings. It takes short time to prepare. You cant eat one just like the potato chips.
Prep time: 12 minutes | Total Prep & Cooking Time: 50 minutes | Servings: 12

Ingredients:
For the cake:
- 2/3 cup coconut flour
- 1 ¼ cup monk fruit sweetener, granulated
- 2/3 cup coconut oil, softened
- 1 tsp. baking soda
- 9 large eggs
- ½ tsp. ground cinnamon
- 2 tsp. vanilla extract, sugar-free
- ¾ tsp. xanthan gum
- ½ tsp. salt
- 2 tsp. cream of tartar

For the topping:
- 3 tbsp. coconut flour
- ¼ cup monk fruit sweetener, granulated
- 1 cup coconut, shredded
- 5 tbsp. coconut oil, melted
- 1 ¼ tsp. ground cinnamon

Instructions:
1. Set your stove to the temperature of 350° Fahrenheit. Use butter to liberally lubricate a 9-inch square pan.
2. In a big dish, cream the eggs with an electrical beater. Add the coconut oil and vanilla extract mixing thoroughly.
3. In a separate dish, whisk the sweetener and coconut flour and blend until there are no lumps in the batter.
4. Add in the cinnamon, cream of tartar, xanthan gum and salt until incorporated.
5. Combine slowly all of the ingredients with an electrical beater until the dough forms.
6. Distribute the batter to the prepped cake pan and heat in the stove for 35 minutes.
7. In an additional dish, whisk the sweetener and coconut with an electrical beater until mixed together. Then stir in the coconut oil, cinnamon, and coconut flour until crumbly.
8. Pull the cake out of the stove and move to the counter for 30 minutes to cool in the pan.
9. Apply the crumble topping and slice before serving.

Nutritional Info Per Serving:
Calories 266 | Fat 24.5g | Carbs 7.8g | Protein 5.5g

Cream & Berries Cake

A berry cake is moist, tender and is filled with ripe berries which are suspended in the light. Its one of the easiest recipes and is made with fresh ingredients that are seasonal.
Prep time: 35 minutes | Cooking Time: 35 minutes | Servings: 8 Slices

Ingredients:
For the cake:
- 1¾ cup almond flour
- 2 tsp. baking powder, gluten-free
- 1 cup sweetener, granulated
- 2 tsp. vanilla extract, sugar-free
- 7 large eggs
- ½ tsp. cream of tartar

For the filling:
- 1 cup sweetener, granulated
- 8 oz. cream cheese, softened
- 2 cups mixed berries
- 1 tsp. vanilla extract, sugar-free
- 2 cups heavy whipping cream
- ½ cup raspberries

For the topping:
- 1 cup mixed berries

Instructions:

1. Set your stove to the temperature of 350° Fahrenheit. Cover a jelly roll pan with baking paper or a non-stick mat.
2. In a food processor set on medium/high, cream the vanilla extract, eggs and cream of tartar for 9 minutes.
3. In a big dish, combine the almond flour and sweetener to remove all lumps. Add 1 egg and combine well. Repeat until all eggs are mixed.
4. Blend in the baking powder.
5. Use a rubber scraper to combine the whipped cream. It needs to keep the fluffiness while being incorporated into the batter.
6. Evenly distribute the cake batter in the prepared roll, coating to the edges with a rubber scraper. Heat in the stove for 20 – 22 minutes.
7. Place a tea towel on top of a wire rack. Straight after the cake is taken out of the stove, take a blunt edge to slice along the cake to make sure it is not stuck to the pan. Turn the cake upside down onto the tea towel and remove the pan.
8. Using the tea towel, roll the cake in a circle and tie the tea towel around it to keep it in place while it cools. Leave to the side while making the filling and whipped cream.
9. In the food processor set on medium, cream the vanilla extract, sweetener, and cream cheese until there are no lumps present. Add in the raspberries and stir, crushing them into the batter.
10. In an additional bowl, cream the heavy whipping cream on high with an electrical beater for 4 minutes.
11. Use a rubber scraper to combine the cream cheese and whipping cream and beat again for 30 seconds.
12. Once the cake has cooled, carefully unroll to evenly distribute the filling over the entire cake. Shake the mixed berries on top of the filling and use the tea towel to roll back into place.
13. Put the rolled cake onto a serving plate and sprinkle the rest of the mixed berries on top. Slice and serve.

Nutritional Info Per Serving:
Calories 441 | Fat 37.2g | Carbs 13.3g | Protein 13.9g

Chocolate Bonbons

These delicious and beautiful bonbons are very easy to make and great for any time of the day.
Prep time: 2 hours | Servings: 6
Ingredients:
- 5 tbsps. Butter
- 3 tbsps. Coconut oil
- 2 tbsps. Sugar-free raspberry syrup
- 2 tbsps. Cocoa powder

Instructions:
1. Mix the entire batch of ingredients in a pan.
2. Empty the bombs into six molds or muffin tins.
3. Place the prepared tin into the freezer for a minimum of two hours. Enjoy!

Nutritional Info Per Serving:
Calories164 | Fat 14.7g | Carbs 7.7g | Protein 3.2g

Chocolate Coconut Bites

These chocolate bites are very sweet and look like truffles. They are very easy to make.
Prep time: 2 hours | Cooking Time: | Servings: 6
Ingredients:
- 4 oz. Unsweetened 80% or higher dark chocolate
- 1/3 cup Heavy cream
- 1 cup Coconut flour
- 1 tbsp. Chocolate protein powder
- ¼ cup Shredded unsweetened coconut
- 4 tbsps. Coconut oil

Instructions:
1. Dice the dark chocolate into bits.
2. Warm up the heavy cream in a saucepan (med-low). Stir in the chocolate bits and oil. Continue stirring until combined and remove from the burner.
3. Stir in the protein powder and coconut flour. Store in the refrigerator for a minimum of two hours.
4. Take the dough out of the fridge when they are cool. Shape into balls and roll through the shredded coconut until coated.
5. Store in the fridge in a closed container.

Nutritional Info Per Serving:

Calories 237 | Fat 18.5g | Carbs 19.7g | Protein 5.5g

Chocolate Covered Almonds

These almonds are salty and very sweet. They are made with almonds that have been coated in chocolate that has melted and then top with sea salt. It is usually ready in few minutes.

Prep time: 10 minutes | Cooking Time: 30 minutes | Servings: 1

Ingredients:
- ¾ cup Unsweetened dark chocolate baking chips
- 1.5 cups Whole raw almonds
- 1 tsp. Pure vanilla extract
- 1 pinch Sea salt

Instructions:
1. Cut a piece of parchment paper and cover a baking tray.
2. Toss the chips into a saucepan using low heat. Stir and add the vanilla.
3. Once the chocolate is melted, add the almonds and stir until coated.
4. Arrange them on the baking tin and dust with the salt.
5. Place in the fridge for a minimum of 30 minutes before you are ready to devour your portion.
6. For a taste change, sprinkle with some ground cinnamon.

Nutritional Info Per Serving:
Calories 1482 | Fat 120g | Carbs 27.5g | Protein 33g

Almond Joy

This dessert is very yummy and includes coconut oil, sugar, sweet coconut and some dark chocolate. For a better treat, you can top with more chocolate and almonds.

Prep Time: 45 minutes | Cooking Time: 15 minutes | Servings: 6

Ingredients
- 8 ounces brown rice syrup
- 8 ounces shredded coconut
- 8 ounces dark chocolate chips
- ½ cup almonds or any nut of your choice, raw or dry roasted

Instructions:
1. Combine the shredded coconut together with the syrup in a medium-sized bowl; mix well until the coconut clumps together, for a couple of minutes.
2. Make small candies from the mixture & place an almond in middle of each one.
3. Now, melt the chocolate in a microwave or double boiler.
4. Dip each candy into the chocolate & arrange it onto wax paper.
5. Put the coated candies into a freezer and let chill until set.
6. Serve and enjoy.

Nutritional Info Per Serving:
Calories 428 | Fat 20.1g | Carbs 23.2g | Protein 4.4g

Candy Dots

You can make great candy dots with just few ingredients. Its for recreating childhood memories and is also for putting a smile of the kid's face.

Prep Time: 15 minutes | Cooking Time: 2 hours & 45 minutes | Servings: 4

Ingredients
- cups allulose
- ¼ cup pasteurized egg white
- Food coloring

Instructions:
1. Using a hand-mixer; whisk the egg white for a minute or two, until completely frothy.
2. Slowly add in the allulose; continue to whisk until peaks form.
3. Evenly divide the prepared mixture into bowls as many as you want to color.
4. Slowly add the drops of color to each bowl until you achieve your desired color.
5. Mix until the color is uniform and then transfer each color to a zippered sandwich bag.
6. Print template & place under each paper you will be piping onto. Clip a very small tip off of one corner of each bag and pipe dots onto unprinted sheets.
7. Let set for a couple of hours and then cut the strips apart.

Nutritional Info Per Serving:
Calories195 | Fat 3.5g | Carbs 9g| Protein 26g

Lemon Cheesecake Mousse

This lemon mouse is a great summer dessert. Its light, soft and delicious.

Prep time: 1 hour 10 minutes | Servings: 5

Ingredients:
- 4 oz. of heavy whipping cream
- ½ tsp. liquid Stevia, lemon flavored
- 8 oz. cream cheese
- 1/8 tsp. salt
- 4 tbsp. lemon juice

Instructions:
1. Using a food processor on high, whisk the heavy whipping cream for 4 minutes.
2. In a dish, whip the cream cheese and lemon juice with an electric blender.
3. Add the mixture to the food processor and whip on high for 2 additional minutes.
4. Taste test the mousse and add more sweetener to taste.
5. Spoon the mousse into a pastry bag and pipe into serving glasses.
6. Dust the tops with lemon zest and cool in the refrigerator for 1 hour before serving.

Nutritional Info Per Serving:
Calories 239 | Fat 24.3g | Carbs 2.1g | Protein 4g

English Custard

Prep time: 10 minutes | Cooking Time: 25 minutes | Servings: 2

Ingredients
- 1½ tsp. Caramel sauce
- 1 cup water
- 1½ Tbsp. allulose
- 2 oz. Cream

Instructions:
1. Take out a blender and place the eggs, cream cheese, water, caramel sauce, and allulose and blend everything together well.
2. Pour this into a heat proof bowl that is going to fit well inside your Instant Pot.
3. Pour a cup of water into the Instant Pot and place the bowl into the steamer basket inside the pot.
4. Add the lid on top and use your Steam function for this one. Cook for the next 20 minutes.
5. After this time, let the pressure out quickly before serving.

Nutritional Info Per Serving:
Calories 86 | Fat 6.3g | Carbs 6.9g | Protein 1g

Pumpkin Cheesecake Mousse

This is a fluffy and super light dessert. Its packed with spices and has enough sweetness to balance the flavor of the pumpkin.

Prep time: 1 hour 15 minutes | Servings: 10

Ingredients:
- ¾ cup heavy whipping cream
- 15 oz. pumpkin puree, unsweetened
- 2 tbsp. pumpkin pie spice
- 12 oz. cream cheese, softened
- 2 tsp. vanilla extract, sugar-free
- ½ cup allulose

Instructions:
1. Using a food processor set on high, whisk the pumpkin puree and cream cheese for 5 minutes.
2. Combine the heavy whipping cream, pumpkin pie spice, vanilla extract, and allulose until creamy.
3. Spoon the mousse into a pastry bag and pipe into serving cups.
4. Refrigerate for 1 hour before serving.

Nutritional Info Per Serving:
Calories 170 | Fat 15.5g | Carbs 5.5g | Protein 3.3g

Cheesecake Pudding

This pudding is really good and is meant to be savoured and nibbled in small and little bites.

Prep time: 10 minutes | Servings: 6

Ingredients:
- 1 block Cream cheese
- ½ cup Heavy whipping cream
- 1 tsp. Lemon juice
- ½ cup Sour cream
- 20 drops Liquid stevia
- 1 tsp. Vanilla extract

Instructions:
1. Microwave the cream cheese for 30 seconds or leave on the counter to soften for a few minutes before using.
2. Whip the sour cream and whipping cream together with a hand mixer until soft peaks form. Combine with the rest of the fixings and whip until fluffy.
3. Portion into four dishes to chill. Cover with plastic wrap in the fridge.

Nutritional Info Per Serving:
Calories 138 | Fat 13.7g | Carbs 2.5g | Protein 2.2g

Coconut Lemon Custard Pie

This pie is keto friendly and very low in carbs. It doesn't require making a crust for it to be a crustless pie.

Prep time: 10 minutes | Cooking time: 45 minutes | Servings: 8

Ingredients:
- ¼ cup coconut flour
- 1 tsp lemon zest
- 2 large eggs
- 1 tsp vanilla extract
- 1 cup coconut milk, canned
- ¾ tsp baking powder
- ¾ cup erythritol
- 4 ounces unsweetened shredded coconut
- 2 tbsp unsalted butter, melted
- ½ tsp lemon extract

Instructions:
1. Preheat oven to 350°F and get a 9-inch pie dish ready by spraying it with cooking spray.
2. Take a large mixing bowl, add coconut flour, lemon zest, eggs, vanilla extract, coconut milk, baking powder and mix together all the ingredients.
3. Add lemon extract, butter and erythritol to the mixture and mix well until combined. Fold the unsweetened shredded coconut in the mixture.
4. Transfer the prepared mixture to the pie dish.
5. Place in the preheated oven and bake for 45 minutes or until you see that the top is golden brown and the edges are full brown.
6. Remove from the oven once baked properly and allow to cool.
7. Cut into triangular pieces and enjoy the amazing lemon coconut custard pie.

Nutritional Info Per Serving:
Calories 240 | Fat 17.9g | Carbs 34.8g | Protein 5.3g

Chapter 9: Cookies & Candy

Fifth Avenue Candy

Sweet candies for any time
Prep Time: 30 minutes | Cooking Time: 30 minutes | Servings: 10

Ingredients
- 1 cup allulose
- 10 ounces peanut butter
- ⅔ cup corn syrup
- Butter & swerve as required to coat pan
- 1 cup water

Instructions:
1. Lightly grease a 10" or 12" skillet with some butter.
2. Mound the peanut butter in middle of your skillet.
3. Coat a large-sized cookie sheet with swerve (enough to cover).
4. Combine corn syrup together with allulose and water in a large pot or saucepan.
5. Cook until it reaches the hard crack on a candy thermometer.
6. Pour the mixture on top of peanut butter; give everything a good.
7. Pour the mixture immediately over the prepared cookie sheet.
8. Immediately roll out to ½" to ¼" thickness.
9. Using a pizza cutter; cut it into desired rectangles.
10. Let completely cool.
11. Coat with the tempered chocolate or melted candy coating.

Nutritional Info Per Serving:
Calories 719 | Fat 44.1g | Carbs 17.8g | Protein 11g

Chocolate Chip Cookies

These have chewy middles and the edges are crispy.
Prep time: 7 minutes | Cooking Time: 15 minutes | Servings: 24

Ingredients:
- ½ tsp. Molasses – optional
- 1 Large egg
- 2/3 cup swerve
- 5.5 tbsps. butter– room temperature
- ½ tsp. Vanilla extract
- 1¼ cups Almond flour
- 1/8 tsp Sea salt
- 1.5 tsp. Baking powder
- 1 tbsp. Coconut flour
- ¼ cup Chopped pecans
- ½ cup Chocolate chips

Instructions:
1. Use some parchment paper or silicone baking mats to line two baking sheets. Set the oven temperature to 325ºF. Use a mixer to blend the sweetener and butter. Mix in the molasses, egg, and vanilla extract until well combined.
2. In another container, combine the two flours, sea salt, and baking powder, stirring until blended.
3. Fold in the pecans and chocolate chips. Arrange the cookie dough by the tablespoonful into the prepared pans. They should be 1.5-inches apart.
4. Bake until the bottoms are browned or about 12-15 minutes. Let them cool until firm and set (minimum 25 minutes).

Nutritional Info Per Serving:
Calories 69 | Fat 5.1g | Carbs 10.9g | Protein 2.1g

Chocolate Coconut Cookies

Nothing beats Chocolate Coconut Cookies when taken as breakfast. They have a unique texture and mouth feel. It is tastefully crunchy to every bit
Prep time: 8 minutes | Cooking Time: 20 minutes | Servings: 20

Ingredients:
- 1 cup Almond flour
- 3 tbsps. Coconut flour
- ¼ tsp. Salt
- 1/3 cup Unsweetened shredded coconut
- 1/3 cup Erythritol
- ½ tsp. Baking powder
- ¼ cup Cocoa powder
- ¼ cup Coconut oil
- ¼ tsp. Vanilla extract
- 2 eggs

Instructions:
1. Warm up the oven to 350ºF. Cover a baking tin with some parchment paper.
2. Combine the dry fixings and mix with a hand mixer.

3. In another dish, combine the wet components and add to the dry until well blended.
4. Break apart pieces of the cookie dough and roll into 20 balls.
5. Arrange on the cookie sheet and bake 15-20 minutes.

Nutritional Info Per Serving:
Calories 54 | Fat 4.7g | Carbs 5.9g | Protein 1.4g

Coconut No-Bake Cookies

These cookies are chocolaty, simple, delicious, perfectly sweet and quick to make.
Chocolaty
Prep time: 10 minutes | Cooking Time: 0 | Servings: 20

Ingredients:
- 1 cup Melted coconut oil
- ½ cup Monk fruit sweetened maple syrup or your favorite
- 3 cups Shredded unsweetened coconut flakes

Instructions:
1. Cut out a sheet of parchment paper and place on a cookie tray.
2. Combine all of the fixings.
3. Run your hands through some water from the tap and shape the mixture into small balls. Arrange them on the pan around one to two inches apart.
4. Press them down to form a cookie and refrigerate until firm.
5. You can prepare these into individual bags if you're an on-the-go kind of person. It will stay fresh covered for up to 7 days (room temperature). Store in the fridge for up to a month or frozen up to two months.

Nutritional Info Per Serving:
Calories 157 | Fat 14.9g | Carbs 7.1g | Protein 0.4g

Cream Cheese Cookies

These fluffy and delicious cream cheese cookies have a very delightful flavor and melt in your mouth. They have a hint of vanilla and a nice tag from the cream cheese.
Prep time: 6 minutes | Cooking Time: 10 minutes | Servings: 4

Ingredients:
- ¾ cup maple syrup or your favorite sugar substitute
- 4 oz. Softened cream cheese
- 1 cup Butter
- 1 Egg
- ½ cup Coconut flour
- 2 cups Almond flour

Instructions:
1. Warm up the oven to 350ºF.
2. Cream the sweetener and butter until fluffy. Fold in the cream cheese and add the egg. Stir in both flours and mix in the vanilla.
3. Chill the prepared dough for a minimum of four hours.
4. Squeeze the dough into a cookie press. You can also roll it into a log and slice.
5. Bake 8-10 minutes – pressed cookies or 10-12 minutes – sliced.

Nutritional Info Per Serving:
Calories 664 | Fat 64.6g | Carbs 32.2g | Protein 7g

Ginger Snap Cookies

These use candied and fresh ginger.
Prep time: 5 | Cooking Time: 11 minutes | Servings: 3

Ingredients:
- ¼ tsp. Ground cloves
- ¼ tsp. Nutmeg
- ¼ tsp. Salt
- 2 cups Almond flour
- ½ tsp. Ground cinnamon
- ¼ cup Unsalted butter
- 1 tsp. Vanilla extract
- 1 Large egg

Instructions:
1. Warm up the oven temperature to 350ºF.
2. Whisk the dry components in a mixing bowl. Blend in the rest of the ingredients into the dry mixture using a hand blender. The dough will be stiff.
3. Measure out the dough for each cookie and flatten with a fork or your fingers.
4. Bake for about 9-11 minutes or until browned.

Nutritional Info Per Serving:
Calories 270 | Fat 26.3g | Carbs 4.8g | Protein 6.1g

Nut Butter Cookies

Easy to make and tasty.

Prep time: 8 | Cooking Time: 12 minutes | Servings: 10
Ingredients:
- 8.8 oz. Almond butter
- ¼ cup Powdered Erythritol
- 1 Egg
- 2½ cups baking flour
- ¼ tsp. Salted butter
- ¼ cup Raw coconut butter

Instructions:
1. Warm up the oven to 320ºF. Prepare a cookie sheet with a sheet of parchment paper.
2. Using a double boiler, melt the almond butter. Take it from the heat and stir in the Erythritol, salt, and egg. Fold until well mixed.
3. Break into 10 segments and roll into balls. Place on the prepared pan and flatten with a fork or your hand.
4. Bake for 12 minutes until browned to your liking.

Nutritional Info Per Serving:
Calories 236 | Fat 12.6g | Carbs 26.1g | Protein 6.9g

Orange Walnut Cookies

These are orange flavoured cookies and are very sweet. Ideal for any time
Prep time: 10 minutes | Cooking Time: 40 minutes | Servings: 10
Ingredients:
- 8 oz. Walnut halves
- 3 tbsp. zested Minced orange
- 1 Eggs
- 20 Stevia drops
- 4 tbsps. Cinnamon – garnish
- 2 tbsps. Shredded coconut – garnish

Instructions:
1. Set the oven temperature to about 320ºF. Toast the walnuts for about 10 minutes until browned. Add them to a food processor. Toss in the rest of the fixings and continue blending until it's smooth.
2. Shape into ten balls and slightly flatten. Drizzle with some shredded coconut.
3. Bake for 40 minutes. Cool on the rack a few minutes and add to a platter to finish cooling. Store in an air-tight container and enjoy any time.

Nutritional Info Per Serving:
Calories 152 | Fat 14g | Carbs 3.4g | Protein 6.1g

Boston Baked Beans Candy

These candies are very sweet, tasty and great when served with honey, biscuits and fresh cornbread.
Prep Time: 20 minutes | Cooking Time: 40 minutes | Servings: 6
Ingredients:
- 2 cup peanuts, raw
- 1 cup allulose
- ½ cup water

Instructions:
1. Place the entire ingredients in a large skillet. Cook over moderate heat until the water is evaporated, stirring every now and then.
2. Pour the mixture on a large-sized cookie sheet and bake in oven for 20 minutes at 325°F. Break apart, if required.

Nutritional Info Per Serving:
Calories 401 | Fat 24g | Carbs 41.2g | Protein 12.6g

Fresh Breath Mints

These mints are very great and leaves the mouth fresh
Servings: 50
Ingredients:
- 1 cup xylitol
- 4 drops peppermint extract

Instructions:
1. In a medium saucepan, melt xylitol at 300 degrees F.
2. Once melted, lower temperature to 275 degrees F and add the peppermint oil.
3. Spread on a silicone baking sheet and let dry for 24 hours.
4. Break the hardened mixture into serving sizes or approximately 1 gram.

Nutritional Info per serving:
Calories 3 | Fats 0 g | Carbs 1 g | Proteins 10 g

Peanut Brittle

Yummy and sweet and require only 3 ingredients to make them
Prep time: 5 minutes | Cooking time: 20 minutes | Servings: 4
Ingredients:
- 1 cup peanuts, salted and roasted
- 2 oz butter

- 3 oz swerve sweetener
- 1 tsp vanilla extract

Instructions:
1. Line a cookie sheet with wax paper and spread out the peanuts.
2. Using a small saucepan over medium heat, combine the butter, sweetener, and vanilla.
3. Cook until it reaches the caramelized stage and is deep brown in color. Do not undercook to avoid making your brittle grainy.
4. Pour the caramel over the spread peanuts and let it cool for 30 minutes to an hour. Once it hardens, break into pieces before serving.

Nutritional Info per serving:
Calories 316 | Fats 29 g | Carbs 5 g | Proteins 10 g

Crystal Candy Skewers

They are sweet and great especially for the kids.
Prep time: 3 hours | Cooking time: - | Servings: 10

Ingredients:
- 4 cups granulated sweetener
- 2 cups water
- 1/2 tsp peppermint extract
- 2 drops green food coloring

Instructions:
1. Wet 10 skewers with water then roll it them in the granulated sugar. Put it aside to dry.
2. Pour the water and bring it to a boil in a medium size pan. Add the granulated sweetener one cup at a time while stirring continuously.
3. Boil until the sweetener dissolves.
4. Remove from heat. Add the peppermint and the green food coloring and stir to get an even color.
5. Allow the syrup to cool down for 10 minutes before pouring into the slim glasses.
6. Dip one skewer per glass, using two clothespins to hold your glass straight and steady. Make sure each skewer hangs an inch from the bottom.
7. Place the glasses in a cool place away from sunlight and cover the top loosely with plastic wrap.
8. After two to four hours, crystals will start to form inside the glass. Allow the crystal to grow until it reaches your desired size. The crystals will expand inside the glass so make sure it does not over grow inside your glass.
9. Crack the crystal gently and pull out the skewer to dry before serving.

Nutritional Info per serving:
Calories 34 | Fats 0 g | Carbs 8 g | Protein: 0 g

Pecan Brittle Squares

These brittles have an awesome taste from nuts and is so sweet. It has a warmth from maple.
Prep time: 25 minutes | Cooking time: - | Servings: 24

Ingredients:
- 12 pieces choc zero chocolate
- 1/2 cup choc zero syrup, caramel
- 1/4 cup unsalted butter
- 4 tbsp monk fruit, powdered
- 2 oz chopped pecans

Instructions:
1. Use half of the pecans to fill each square of your brownie square silicone mold.
2. In a saucepan, melt the butter on low heat. One butter is melted, turn the heat to medium-low heat and add the syrup and monk fruit, whisking frequently.
3. Get it to boiling point and wait for the mixture to froth without forming bubbles. Whisk for 30 seconds then remove from heat before whisking for another 20 seconds.
4. Pour over the silicone mold, filling it halfway.
5. Melt the chocolate on a double boiler.
6. Stir in the chocolate and let it cool for a minute or two before pouring over the silicone mold, covering the caramel.
7. Top the chocolate with the remaining pecans.
8. Let it cool to room temperature before wrapping.
9. Serve as a snack or as dessert.

Nutritional Info per serving:
Calories 63 | Fats 5.4 g | Carbs 10.3 g | Proteins 0.2 g

Brittle Butterscotch Candy

Sweet and so tasty. Filled with lots of flavor

Prep time: 5 minutes | Cooking time: 10 minutes | Servings: 16
Ingredients:
- 1 cup butter, grass-fed
- 1/2 cup monk fruit sweetener
- 1 tsp vanilla extract
- 1 tsp pink Hmalayan salt

Instructions:
1. Using a heavy bottom pan, melt butter over medium heat.
2. Add the sweetener and stir often. Bring to a boil and continue to stir.
3. When the mixture reaches boiling point, reduce heat to low.
4. Continue stirring until the mixture turns amber in color.
5. Remove from the heat and stir in salt and vanilla.
6. Cool for three minutes while stirring.
7. Pour in an 8x8-inch pan and put in the fridge at least 8 hours or overnight.
8. Break into pieces before serving.

Nutritional Info per serving:
Calories 102 | Fats 12 g | Carbs 5 g | Protein: 0 g

Pecan Candies

These candies are a favourite for many people why try them because they are full of sweetness.
Prep time: 8 minutes | Cooking time: 20 minutes | Servings: 24
Ingredients:
- 6 tbsp swerve brown
- 3 tbsp allulose
- 5 tbsp butter
- 1/2 cup heavy cream
- 1/4 tsp xanthan gum
- 1/4 tsp sea salt
- 2 cups pecans, cut in halves
- 4 oz dark chocolate, sugar free, chopped

Instructions:
1. Combine 4 tbsp of butter and the sweeteners on medium heat in a large saucepan.
2. Cook for 3 to 5 minutes or until boiling. Take off of the heat and add the cream. This will make the mixture bubble.
3. Return the mixture to medium heat and wait for boiling point. Boil 3 minutes. Sprinkle the xanthan gum and salt, then whisk.
4. Let cool for an hour. Make sure it is creamy thick and not solid.
5. Preheat the oven at 360 degrees F. Line a cookie tray with wax paper. Spread the out the pecans and toast for 7-10 minutes. After toasting, arrange the pecans in clusters of 3 to 4 pieces.
6. Drizzle each cluster with 2-3 teaspoons of caramel. Make sure there is enough caramel to clump the pecans together. Place the cookie tray in the freezer and let the caramel harden.
7. In a double boiler, combine a tbsp of butter and dark chocolate. Stir until melted and smooth. Top over the chilled pecans.
8. Sprinkle with salt and let set before serving.

Nutritional Info per serving:
Calories 242 | Fats 215 g | Carbs 6.6 g | Proteins 2.4 g

Bourbon Candy Balls

These candies are great and tasty. Try them today.
Prep time: 25 minutes | Cooking time: - | Servings: 20
Ingredients:
- 1/2 cup pecans, chopped
- 1/4 cup bourbon
- 1 cup swerve confectioners
- 8 tbsp butter, unsalted and softened
- 2 oz cream cheese, softened
- 2 1/2 tbsp coconut flour
- 3/4 cup dark chocolate, sugar-free
- 2 tsp coconut oil
- 20 pecans, halved

Instructions:
1. Pre-soak 1/2 cup chopped pecans in bourbon for 24 hours.
2. In a mixing bowl, mix with an electric mixer the swerve, butter, and cream cheese until it turns creamy and fluffy.
3. Add the pecan and bourbon mixture and coconut flour and mix until it becomes smooth. Refrigerate for 10 minutes.
4. After chilling, scoop a tbsp of the mixture on a lined baking sheet and shape it into a ball. Freeze the balls in the freezer.

5. While waiting, prepare a double boiler over medium heat and melt the dark chocolate and coconut oil. Stir constantly until completely melted.
6. Remove the bourbon balls in the freezer and dip them one at a time into the melted chocolate. Then place it back on the lined baking sheet and top with one half of the pecan.
7. Return to the freezer and let it set before serving.

Nutritional Info per serving:
Calories 123 | Fats 11 g | Carbs 3 g | Protein: 1 g

Mixed Nuts Choco Candy Clusters

These candies make a great and delicious holiday hostess gift.
Prep time: 5 minutes | Cooking time: 10 minutes | Servings: 25

Ingredients:
- 9 oz dark chocolate chips, sugar-free
- 1/4 cup coconut oil, unrefined
- 2 cups mixed nuts, salted

Instructions:
1. Prepare a silicone-baking mat on a baking tray.
2. On a double boiler, melt chocolate chips. Add coconut oil and stir until well combined. Add the mixed nuts and fold into the chocolate mixture until coated completely.
3. On the baking mat, scoop large spoonful of the chocolate nut mixture. Space them out so they don't stick together.
4. Place in the fridge until it sets and serve.

Nutritional Info per serving:
Calories 170 | Fats 19.9 g | Carbs 5.3 g | Protein 3.2 g

Crispy Cookies

You will definitely love the buttery edges and crackly tops of these cookies. Whe you take a bite, it is so satisfying.
Prep time: 5 minutes | Cooking time: 25 minutes | Servings: 12

Ingredients:
- 2 eggs
- 1 tbsp soy flour
- 3 tbsp almond flour
- 1-2 tsp coconut chips
- 1/2 cup milk
- 1 tsp baking soda
- 1 tsp vanilla extract
- Any sweetener of your choice

Instructions:
1. Prepare the oven by preheating it to 350 degrees F.
2. Place parchment paper over a baking sheet and lay 12 silicone molds on it.
3. Combine all the ingredients together in a large bowl and leave it to stand for 15 minutes.
4. The dough will be a little watery.
5. Pour the dough into the silicone molds and put the baking tray in the oven.
6. Bake the cookies for 20 minutes.
7. Once cooked, remove the cookies from the oven and leave to cool completely before serving them.

Nutritional info per serving:
Calories 104 | Fats 9g | Carbs 11g | Protein 12.3g

Nutty Cookies

So sweet and full of lots of flavors and crunchy
Prep time: 6 minutes | Cooking time: 15 minutes | Servings: 18

Ingredients:
- 1/4 cup coconut oil
- 4 tbsp soft butter
- 2 tbsp swerve
- 4 egg yolks
- 1 cup dark cacao dark chocolate
- 1 cup coconut flakes
- 3/4 cup walnuts roughly chopped

Instructions:
1. Prepare the oven by preheating it to 350 degrees F.
2. Place parchment paper over a baking sheet.
3. Combine the egg yolks, sweetener, butter, coconut oil, walnuts, coconut, and cacao dark chocolate in a large bowl and stir to combine.
4. Spoon the batter out onto the baking tray and bake for 15 minutes.
5. Once cooked, remove from the oven and allow to cool down completely before serving.

Nutritional info per serving:

Calories 135 | Fats 6.3g | Carbs 7.2g | Proteins 4g

Snickerdoodle Cookies

Easy, tasty, fast and sweet with spices
Prep time: 7 minutes | Cooking time: 15 minutes | Servings: 16

Ingredients:
For the cookies:
- 2 cups almond flour, superfine
- 1/2 cup softened salted butter
- A pinch of kosher salt
- 3/4 cup granulated erythritol
- 1/2 tsp baking soda

For the coating:
- 2 tbsp granulated erythritol
- 1 tsp ground cinnamon

Instructions:
1. Prepare the oven by preheating it to 350 degrees F.
2. Place parchment paper over a baking sheet.
3. In a medium sized bowl combine all the cookie ingredients and whisk with an electric mixer until a dough is formed.
4. Use your hands to roll the dough into balls.
5. On a small plate, combine the cinnamon and sweetener.
6. Roll the balls into the mix and arrange them onto the baking tray.
7. Put the cookies into the oven and bake for 15 minutes.
8. Once cooked, remove the tray from the oven and serve.

Nutritional info per serving:
Calories 131 | Fats 13g | Carbs 1.5g | Proteins 3g

Chapter 10: Smoothies

Blueberry and Soy Smoothie

This smoothie is full of good fat, and a great flavor and color! Keep any leftovers in an airtight container in the fridge for up to 24 hours so you can enjoy a quick pick me up later on!

Prep time: 5 minutes | Servings: 2

Ingredients
- 2 cups fresh or frozen red blueberries
- 1-cup nonfat or 1 percent milk
- 2 scoops of vanilla soy protein powder
- 3 Tbsp. red raspberry preServings
- 3 ice cubes (optional)

Instructions:
1. Put all the ingredients in a blender. Cover and blend at high speed.
2. Enjoy.

Nutritional info per serving:
Calories 430 | Carbs 6 g | Fats 2 g | Proteins 34g

Blueberry Avocado Smoothie

This is a filling and yummy smoothie you can have for breakfast or as a quick snack to up your fat intake. It's super low carb and delicious!

Prep time: 3 minutes | Servings: 2

Ingredients:
- 1 cup medium blueberries
- 1 avocado
- 1½-tbsps unsweetened cocoa powder
- ¾- cup frozen raspberries
- 1½-cups almond milk

Instructions:
1. Put all ingredients in a blender and blend on high until smooth.
2. Enjoy!

Nutritional info per serving:
Calories 363 | Fats 24g | Proteins 42g | Carbs 10g

Blackberry Smoothie

This smoothie is definitely full of benefits! Enjoy this smoothie very cold.

Prep time: 5 minutes | Servings: 2

Ingredients
- 0.5 cup of fresh or frozen blackberries
- 1 tbsp lemon juice
- 0.5 tsp vanilla extract
- 14oz coconut milk

Instructions:
1. Add all ingredients into the blender and combine until you get a rich and smooth consistency
2. Pour into your serving glass and add a little more lemon juice if you like

Nutritional info per serving:
Calories 363 | Carbs 12g | Fats 10g | Proteins 34g

Berry Acai Smoothie

This smoothie is refreshing, sweet and fun! When your body adjusts to the keto lifestyle, your taste buds naturally adjust to find foods naturally sweeter.

Prep time: 2 minutes | Servings: 1

Ingredients:
- 1 cup Silk Tofu
- 2 tbsp Coconut Cream
- 1 cup Ice Cubes
- ¼ cup Raspberries
- 2 tbsp Acai Powder
- 3 tbsp Soy Protein Powder

Instructions:
1. Combine all ingredients in a blender.
2. Blend until smooth.

Nutritional info per serving:
Calories 556 | Carbs 10 g | Fats 20 g | Protein 18 g

Choco-Coco Milk Shake

Easy to prepare and super yummy

Prep time: 5 minutes |Servings: 1

Ingredients:
- ½ cup whole milk
- 1 tbsp cocoa powder
- 1 packet Stevia, or more to taste
- 1 tbsp coconut flakes, unsweetened
- 1 cup water
- 1 tbsp coconut oil

Instructions:
1. Add all ingredients in blender.
2. Blend until smooth and creamy.
3. Serve and enjoy.

Nutritional info per serving:

Calories 263 | Carbs 22.7g | Proteins 4.8g | Fats 20.65g

Nutty Choco Milk Shake

This milk shake is exotic and delicious!
Prep time: 5 minutes | Servings: 1
Ingredients:
- ¼ cup whole milk
- 1 tbsp cocoa powder
- 1 packet Stevia, or more to taste
- ¼ cup pecans
- 1 ½ cups water
- 1 tbsp macadamia oil

Instructions:
1. Add all ingredients in blender.
2. Blend until smooth and creamy.
3. Serve and enjoy.

Nutritional info per serving:
Calories 358 | Carbs 15.5g | Proteins 5.1g | Fats 34.0g

Choco Milk Smoothie

This chocolate smoothie is so thick and creamy. Enjoy it extra cold to really get a satisfying experience!
Prep time: 4 minutes | Servings: 1
Ingredients:
- ¼ cup whole milk
- 1 tbsp cocoa powder
- 1 packet Stevia, or more to taste
- 1 tbsp chia seeds
- 1 tbsp hemp seeds
- 1 tbsp flaxseed
- 1 ½ cups water
- 1 tbsp Flaxseed oil

Instructions:
1. Add all ingredients in blender.
2. Blend until creamy yet still gritty. If preferred, blend until smooth.
3. Serve and enjoy.

Nutritional info per serving:
Calories 363 | Carbs 22.8g | Proteins 8.9g | Fats 29.4g

Creamy Choco Shake

This creamy choco shake is the perfect thing to jump start your day!
Prep time: 4 minutes | Servings: 1
Ingredients:
- ½ cup heavy cream
- 2 tbsps cocoa powder
- 1 packet Stevia, or more to taste
- 1 cup water

Instructions:
1. Add all ingredients in blender.
2. Blend until smooth and creamy.
3. Serve and enjoy.

Nutritional info per serving:
Calories 435 | Carbs 10.6g | Proteins 4.6g | Fats 45.5g

Baby Kale and Yogurt Smoothie

Keto smoothies are having their moment in the spotlight, and it's easy to see why! Creamy, thick and delicious, they are the perfect treat for snacking or breakfast!
Prep time: 4 minutes | Servings: 1
Ingredients:
- 1 cup whole milk yogurt
- 1 cup baby kale greens
- 1 packet Stevia, or more to taste
- 1 tbsp MCT oil
- 1 tbsp sunflower seeds
- 1 cup water

Instructions:
1. Add all ingredients in blender.
2. Blend until smooth and creamy.
3. Serve and enjoy.

Nutritional info per serving:
Calories 329 | Carbs 15.6g | Proteins 11.0g | Fats 26.2g

Nutty Arugula Yogurt Smoothie

This nutty smoothie bowl is decadently delicious and full of good fat to fuel your morning!
Prep time: 4 minutes | Servings: 1
Ingredients:
- 1 cup whole milk yogurt
- 1 cup baby arugula
- 1 packet Stevia, or more to taste
- 1 tbsp avocado oil
- 2 tbsps macadamia nuts
- 1 cup water

Instructions:
1. Add all ingredients in blender.
2. Blend until smooth and creamy.
3. Serve and enjoy.

Nutritional info per serving:
Calories 399 | Carbs 15.5g | Proteins 10.3g | Fats 34.8g

Hazelnut-Lettuce Yogurt Shake

This vibrant green shake is just the thing to get you going in the morning! Its a great way to supplement your diet.
Prep time: 4 minutes | Servings: 1
Ingredients:
- 1 cup whole milk yogurt
- 1 cup lettuce chopped
- 1 packet Stevia, or more to taste
- 1 tbsp olive oil
- 3 tbsps Hazelnut chopped
- 1 cup water

Instructions:
1. Add all ingredients in blender.
2. Blend until smooth and creamy.
3. Serve and enjoy.

Nutritional info per serving:
Calories 412 | Carbs 17.2g | Proteins 12.5g | Fats 34.7g

Garden Greens & Yogurt Shake

Sweet and so tasty. It's a great sensation
Prep time: 4 minutes | Servings: 1
Ingredients:
- 1 cup whole milk yogurt
- 1 cup Garden greens
- 1 packet Stevia, or more to taste
- 1 tbsp MCT oil
- 1 tbsp flaxseed, ground
- 1 cup water

Instructions:
1. Add all ingredients in blender.
2. Blend until smooth and creamy.
3. Serve and enjoy.

Nutritional info per serving:
Calories 334 | Carbs 17.2g | Proteins 11.2g | Fats 26.0g

Ginger-Spiced Coconut-Milk Shake

This ginger flavourful shake is the perfect thing if you're craving something a bit different
Prep time: 4 minutes | Servings: 1
Ingredients:
- 1 cup coconut milk
- ½ tsp ginger powder or more to taste
- 1 small stalk celery
- 1 cup Spring mix salad
- 1 tsp sesame seeds
- 1 cup water
- 1 packet Stevia, optional

Instructions:
1. Add all ingredients in blender.
2. Blend until smooth and creamy.
3. Serve and enjoy.

Nutritional info per serving:
Calories 475 | Carbs 10.1g | Proteins 6.1g | Fats 50.0g

Strawberry Coconut Shake

Coconut and strawberries come together in this simple smoothie
Prep time: 4 minutes | Servings: 1
Ingredients:
- ½ cup coconut milk
- 1 ½ cups water
- ½ cup chopped strawberries
- 1 tbsp hemp seeds
- 1 tbsp coconut oil

Instructions:
1. Add all ingredients in blender.
2. Blend until smooth and creamy.
3. Serve and enjoy.

Nutritional info per serving:
Calories 418 | Carbs 11.3g | Proteins 4.7g | Fats 42.5g

Hazelnut and Coconut Shake

Creamy, tasty, and oh-so-satisfying! This shake is the perfect midday snack for a busy day!
Prep time: 4 minutes | Servings: 1
Ingredients:
- ½ cup coconut milk
- ¼ cup hazelnut, chopped
- 1 ½ cups water
- 1 packet Stevia, optional

Instructions:
1. Add all ingredients in blender.
2. Blend until smooth and creamy.
3. Serve and enjoy.

Nutritional info per serving:
Calories 457 | Carbs 12.5g | Protein 7.05g | Fats 46.1g

Cardamom-Cinnamon Spiced Coco-Latte

Try this latte for a wonderful taste and enjoy it
Prep time: 4 minutes | Servings: 1
Ingredients:
- ½ cup coconut milk
- ¼ tsp cardamom powder
- ¼ tsp cinnamon
- ¼ tsp nutmeg

- 1 tbsp chocolate powder
- 1 ½ cups brewed coffee, chilled
- 1 tbsp coconut oil

Instructions:
1. Add all ingredients in blender.
2. Blend until smooth and creamy.
3. Serve and enjoy.

Nutritional info per serving:
Calories 362 | Carbs 7.5g | Proteins 3.8g | Fats 38.7g

Hazelnut-Mocha Shake

This shake will cheer you up greatly
Prep time: 4 minutes | Servings: 1
Ingredients:
- 1 oz hazelnuts
- 2 cups brewed coffee, chilled
- 2 tbsp cocoa powder
- 1-2 packets Stevia, optional
- 1 tbsp MCT oil

Instructions:
1. Add all ingredients in blender.
2. Blend until smooth and creamy.
3. Serve and enjoy.

Nutritional info per serving:
Calories 324 | Carbs 12.0g | Proteins 6.8g | Fats 32.4g

Fruity Morning Smoothie

This recipe is restaurant quality, and so easy to prepare! Take it on its own for a luxuriously simple snack, dinner or anytime.
Prep time: 4 minutes | Servings: 1
Ingredients:
- 3 medium blackberries, whole
- 2 tbsps chopped pecans
- 1 tbsp hemp seeds
- 1 tbsp sunflower seeds
- 1 tbsp coconut flakes, unsweetened
- 2 cups water
- 1 cup Spring mix salad blend
- 1 tbsp avocado oil
- 1 packet Stevia, optional

Instructions:
1. Add all ingredients in blender.
2. Blend until smooth and creamy.
3. Serve and enjoy.

Nutritional info per serving:
Calories 385 | Carbs 16.8g | Proteins 6.9g | Fats 34.8g

Creamy Wake-Me-Up Smoothie

This satisfying smoothie is a great snack or breakfast option! Its full of taste, great texture and flavor!
Prep time: 4 minutes | Servings: 1
Ingredients:
- 2 cups brewed coffee
- ½ avocado fruit
- 1 tsp chia seeds
- 1 tbsp pumpkin seeds
- 1 tbsp sunflower seeds
- 1-2 packets Stevia, optional
- 1 cup Baby Kale salad mix
- 1 tbsp avocado oil

Instructions:
1. Place hot brewed coffee, chia seeds, pumpkin seeds, and sunflower seeds in a bowl or large mug. Let seeds soak in liquid cooled to room temperature. Then chill in fridge.
2. An hour or two later, add all ingredients in blender.
3. Blend until smooth and creamy.
4. Serve and enjoy.

Nutritional info per serving:
Calories 417 | Carbs 16.6g | Proteins 8.3g | Fats 38.9g

Chocolate-Coconut Shake

This shake will keep you full and satisfied for hours! It's really good for you and really delicious, too.
Prep time: 4 minutes | Servings: 1
Ingredients:
- 2 tbsps coconut flakes shredded and unsweetened
- 1 cup pecans
- 2 cups water
- 2 tbsps chocolate powder, unsweetened
- 1-2 packets Stevia, optional
- 1 tbsp avocado oil

Instructions:
1. Add all ingredients in blender.
2. Blend until smooth and creamy.
3. Serve and enjoy.

Nutritional info per serving:
Calories 408 | Carbs 17.4g | Proteins 4.9g | Fats 38.4g

Chapter 11: This & That

Almond Pumpkin Pudding

This dairy free pudding is easy to make and leaves you satisfied and happy.

Prep time: 1 hour 10 minutes | Cooking time: 10 minutes | Servings: 10

Ingredients:
- 5 oz. Coconut oil
- 10 oz. Pumpkin puree
- 5 oz. Coconut cream
- 1 tbsp. Pumpkin pie spice
- 3 tbsp. Powdered Erythritol
- 4 oz. Almonds
- ¾ tsp. Ginger

Instructions:
1. Combine and stir all of the fixings (omit the almonds) in a saucepan on medium heat.
2. Pour into silicone molds and press an almond inside each one.
3. Freeze for a minimum of one hour. Then you can remove from the molds and serve or freeze for later.
4. For a taste change, just squeeze a little lemon juice over the pudding before serving.

Nutritional Info Per Serving:
Calories 235 | Fats 23.4g | Carbs 7.5g | Protein 3.1g

Chocolate Avocado Pudding

The ingredients for making this pudding are simple and its very delicious. There are many substitutes like spices, liquid, sweeteners and its varies in taste.

Prep time: 40 minutes | Servings: 2

Ingredients:
- 2 oz. Room temperature cream cheese
- 1 medium avocado
- 1 tsp. swerve
- ¼ tsp Vanilla extract
- 4 tbsp. Unsweetened cocoa powder
- ¼ tsp Pink salt

Instructions:
1. Combine the cream cheese with the avocado, sweetener, vanilla, cocoa powder, and salt. Add to a blender or processor.
2. Pulse until creamy smooth.
3. Measure into a fancy dessert dishes and chill for at least 30 minutes.

Nutritional Info Per Serving:
Calories 332 | Fats 30.9g | Carbs 16.4g | Proteins 6g

Butter Tossed Asparagus

The old adage is true - butter DOES make it better! This asparagus dish is loaded with delicious fat and flavor and makes the perfect dish.

Prep time: 5 minutes | Cooking Time: 15 minutes | Servings: 2

Ingredients:
- 10 spears fresh asparagus
- 2 Tablespoons butter
- 1 Tablespoon olive oil
- 2 large stems thyme
- 1 teaspoon salt
- 1 teaspoon white pepper

Instructions:
1. Bring a large pot of salted water to a boil. Toss in the asparagus spears, and boil for 1 minute to blanch.
2. Drain, and transfer to an ice bath. Set aside. Preheat a large pan over medium heat.
3. Drizzle in the oil and add the butter and whole thyme stem. Cook until the butter has melted fully and has started to foam, about 2 minutes. Add the blanched asparagus spears to the foaming butter, and toss well to coat. Cook for 1-2 minutes, tossing well the entire time.
4. Serve immediately.

Nutritional info per serving:
Calories 186 | Carbs 2 g | Fats 18.7 g | Proteins 2.8 g

Caramelized Onions

These caramelized onions are low carb, relatively high fat, and make a great addition to pizzas, burgers, or anything else you can come up with.

Prep time: 10 minutes | Cooking Time: 65 minutes | Servings: 8

Ingredients:
- 4 onions, sliced thinly
- 1/2 lb. butter
- 1 Tablespoon salt

Instructions:

1. Melt the butter in a pan over medium heat. Add in the onions and the salt.
2. Toss well with tongs until the onions start to cook down. Continue to cook, stirring occasionally, for about an hour, until the onions are brown and soft.
3. Transfer to an airtight container and keep in the fridge for up to 4 weeks.

Nutritional info per serving:
Calories 225 | Carbs 3 g | Fats 23.1 g | Proteins 0.9 g

Curry Mayonnaise

Curry Mayo is a great option to mix up flavors! Use this mayo on burgers or in the Egg Salad or Chicken Salad as a substitute.
Prep time: 5 minutes | Cooking Time: 0 minutes | Servings: 8

Ingredients:
- 1/4 cup mayonnaise
- 1 Tablespoon curry powder

Instructions:
1. Whisk ingredients together until smooth. Store in an airtight container for up to 5 weeks.

Nutritional info per serving:
Calories 45 | Carbs 0 g | Fats 5 g | Proteins 2 g

Green Tahini

This tahini is enhanced with greens for additional nutritional value and a hit of color! Use this sauce as a dip for veggies, a dressing for salads, or as a replacement for mayo.
Prep time: 5 minutes | Cooking Time: 40 minutes | Servings: 6

Ingredients:
- 2 Tablespoons tahini paste
- 2 cloves garlic
- 2 teaspoons salt
- 1 Tablespoon olive oil
- 1 lemon, juice and zest
- 1/4 cup water
- 1/4 cup fresh kale

Instructions:
1. In a blender or food processor, combine all ingredients until smooth. Taste and adjust seasoning as needed. Store in an airtight container for up to a month.

Nutritional info per serving:
Calories 43 | Carbs 0.3 g | Fats 3.9 g | Proteins 0.7 g

Cheesy Fondue

Fondue is one of the best snacks for sharing. By using low carb veggies like celery and red peppers, you and your friends! can enjoy this high fat, low carb treat.
Prep time: 10 minutes | Cooking Time: 30 minutes | Servings: 4

Ingredients
- 1 cup cheddar cheese, shredded
- 1 cup gruyere cheese, shredded
- 1/4 cup dry white wine
- 1 cup heavy cream
- 1 teaspoon garlic powder
- 1 teaspoon salt
- 1 teaspoon cayenne (optional)
- 3 stalks celery, chopped into 12 equal sticks
- 1/2 red bell pepper, sliced into 8 thin strips
- 4 pickles, cut in half lengthwise

Instructions:
2. In a medium sized saucepan, melt the cheeses and wine together over medium heat. Stir in the cream and spices, mixing well to combine.
3. Transfer the finished sauce to a fondue pot, and keep warm. Arrange the veggies and bread onto a plate.
4. Using fondue forks, dip the veggies into the cheese sauce and eat immediately.

Nutritional info per serving:
Calories 376 | Carbs 4.4 g | Fats 32 g | Proteins 19.5 g

Green Bean Fries

Have a craving for fries, but no potatoes on the Keto Diet, so what do you do? Try these delicious green bean fries smothered in a cheesy herbed mixture. Yummy!
Prep time: 10 minutes | Cooking Time: 10 minutes | Servings: 4

Ingredients
- 24 green beans
- 1 egg
- 1/2 cup parmesan
- 1 teaspoon garlic powder
- 1 teaspoon Italian herbs
- 1 teaspoon salt

Instructions:

1. Preheat oven to 400F. Fill a small pot with water up to three quarters. Bring the water to a boil.
2. Blanch the beans for 2 minutes, and immediately drain and transfer them to an ice bath.
3. Next, beat the egg in one bowl, and combine the dry ingredients in another bowl. Prepare a baking sheet lined with parchment.
4. Bread each bean by dipping it first into the egg, then into the cheese mixture.
5. Lay the prepared beans on the baking sheet, and bake for 15 minutes until crispy.
6. Store any leftover beans in an airtight container at room temperature, and enjoy within 4 days.

Nutritional info per serving:
Calories 113 | Carbs 2 g | Fats 6 g | Proteins 9 g

Celery and Almond Butter

There are many wonderful flavors and textures in this simple and easy snack! The crispy green crunch of celery pairs perfectly with creamy nutty almond butter.
Prep time: 2 minutes | Cooking Time: 0 minutes | Servings: 1

Ingredients
- 2 stalks celery
- 2 Tablespoons almond butter

Instructions
1. Cut the celery into 8 equal sized sticks and dip into the almond butter. For a more portable snack, spread the almond butter into the cavity of the celery stalk, and pack in an airtight container for up to 24 hours.

Nutritional info per serving:
Calories 230 | Carbs 4 g | Fats 18 g | Proteins 8 g

Salted Macadamias

Nuts are a great way to get a quick dose of fat. These nuts are so easy to do, and so delicious! Once you've figured out the basic recipe, it's easy to season these nuts with any herbs or spices.
Prep time: 5 minutes | Cooking Time: 5 minutes | Servings: 1

Ingredients
- 1/4 cup Macadamia nuts
- 1 Tablespoon coconut oil
- 1 teaspoon sea salt

Instructions
2. Preheat oven to 350F. Toss the macadamia nuts in the oil and salt.
3. Lay onto a baking sheet, and bake 5 minutes, making sure not to burn the nuts. Allow to cool fully.

Nutritional info per serving:
Calories 224 | Carbs 1 g | Fats 22 g | Proteins 3 g

Almond Butter Fat Bombs

With a nutty flavor and lots of good fats, these Fat Bombs are one bite snacks you'll really enjoy. You'll need mini muffin tins or muffin cups to make these!
Prep time: 5 minutes | Cooking Time: 0 minutes | Servings: 6

Ingredients:
- 1/4 cup almond butter
- 1/4 cup coconut oil
- 2 Tablespoons cocoa powder
- 1/4 cup Stevia or erythritol

Instructions:
1. With a mixer or by hand, mix together the almond butter and a coconut oil. Microwave for about 30-45 seconds to soften, then stir until smooth.
2. Add the cocoa powder and the sweetener, then stir those in and mix well. Pour into either silicone or mini muffin tins lined with papers.
3. Stick in the fridge until firm.

Nutritional info per serving:
Calories 189 | Carbs 1.4 g | Fats 19.1 g | Proteins 3.2 g

Tahini Sauce

Tahini Sauce is a flavor-packed sauce made with sesame paste. This thick, creamy, dairy free sauce is the perfect dip for veggies, but can also be used as a dressing in lettuce wraps, a sauce for meat, or salad dressing!
Prep time: 10 minutes | Cooking Time: 40 minutes | Servings: 2

Ingredients:
- 1 Tablespoon tahini paste
- 1 teaspoon chopped parsley
- 1 Tablespoon lemon juice
- 1/4 cup water
- 1/2 Tablespoon salt

- 1 clove garlic
- 1/4 cup olive oil
- 1/2 cucumber, cut into 8 equal pieces
- 1 stalk celery, cut into 8 equal pieces

Instructions:
1. In a blender or food processor, combine the tahini, parsley, lemon juice, water, salt, garlic and oil until smooth. Transfer to an airtight container, and store in the fridge for up to two weeks. Serve with veggie sticks.

Nutritional info per serving:
Calories 555 | Carbs 8 g | Fats 58.5 g | Proteins 4 g

Baked Brie

This baked Brie recipe is savory, comforting, and nice for special occasions. For added decadence, serve with Nordic seed bread and sliced low carb veggies like celery, cucumber, or peppers.

Prep time: 5 minutes | Cooking Time: 10 minutes | Servings: 2

Ingredients:
- 6 oz Brie cheese
- 1/2 oz walnuts
- 1/2 oz pine nuts
- 1/2 oz pecans
- 1 clove garlic, minced
- 2 teaspoons smoked paprika
- 4 stems thyme
- 1 Tablespoon salt
- 1 Tablespoon pepper
- 1 Tablespoon olive oil

Instructions:
2. Preheat the oven to 375F. In a medium sized bowl, combine the nuts, garlic, herbs, paprika, salt, pepper and oil.
3. Lay the cheese onto a baking sheet lined with parchment, and spoon the nut mixture over top, so it completely covers the cheese.
4. Bake for 10 minutes, until the cheese is melted and the nuts are fragrant and toasted.
5. Any unfinished cheese can be wrapped and kept in the fridge for up to a month.

Nutritional info per serving:
Calories 501 | Carbs 3.4 g | Fats 44 g | Proteins 21 g

Spicy Mayo

This spicy mayo makes a wonderful burger topper, and is also a great dip for veggies, fried pickles, onion rings, or anything else you can think of! Make a big batch and keep in the fridge!

Prep time: 10 minutes | Cooking Time: 10 minutes | Servings: 12

Ingredients:
- 3 cups mayonnaise
- 6 Tablespoons hot sauce or sriracha

Instructions:
1. Whisk the two ingredients together until smooth. Keep in the fridge for up to 8 weeks.

Nutritional info per serving:
Calories 90 | Carbs 1 g | Fats 10 g | Proteins 0 g

Raspberry Chia Pudding

Chia pudding is so versatile, and really easy to prep in advance! Because chia seeds get better as they expand in liquid, this pudding will continue to thicken and sweeten as it sits in the fridge. The best part is, it's good for up to a week in the fridge.

Prep time: 5 minutes | Cooking Time: 5 minutes | Servings: 2

Ingredients
- 1 cup almond milk
- 1/2 cup chia seeds
- 1/4 cup frozen raspberries
- 1 Tablespoon flaxseeds
- 1 Tablespoon hemp seeds

Instructions
2. Combine all ingredients together, mixing well so the raspberries crush a bit. Store in an airtight container overnight. Enjoy leftovers within 7 days.

Nutritional info per serving:
Calories 642 | Carbs 8 g | Fats 50 g | Proteins 15.9 g

Raspberry Chocolate Fudge

This rich, chocolaty fudge is the perfect thing to hit the spot when you're craving something sweet. Best of all, it's virtually carb and protein free and high fat, which can help kick start your ketosis.

Prep time: 2 minutes | Cooking Time: 10 minutes | Servings: 16

Ingredients
- 1/2 cup raw cacao powder
- 2 Tablespoons unsweetened dark chocolate, shaved
- 2 Tablespoons Stevia
- 1/2 cup coconut oil
- 1/4 cup raspberries, mashed lightly
- 1/4 cup almond milk

Instructions
1. Mix all ingredients together until well combined. Prepare a 10" baking dish with parchment paper or plastic wrap, and carefully spoon the fudge mixture into the center.
2. Using a spatula, spread the mixture evenly into the baking dish, and cover with plastic wrap.
3. Refrigerate for an hour, and cut into 16 equal pieces. Store wrapped in the fridge for up to one month.

Nutritional info per serving:
Calories 74 | Carbs 0.9 g | Fats 8.1 g | Proteins 0.6 g

Strawberry Chia Pudding Popsicles

Popsicles are such a sweet, refreshing treat! These popsicles have extra fat and protein from coconut milk and chia seeds, and are sweetened naturally with fruit.

Prep time: 4 hours | Cooking Time: 0 minutes | Servings: 6

Ingredients
- 2 cups coconut milk
- 1/4 cup chia seeds
- 1/4 cup frozen strawberries, thawed

Instructions
1. Mash together the berries and chia seeds. Stir in the coconut milk. Transfer the mixture to 6 popsicle molds, and freeze for at least 4 hours. Popsicles will last in the freezer for up to 8 weeks.

Nutritional info per serving:
Calories 277 | Carbs 3 g | Fats 24.9 g | Proteins 5 g

Red Pepper Cod

This easy, classic recipe is perfect for a quick weeknight meal! The cooked cod will last for up to a day in the fridge. Serve with sautéed vegetables, a salad, or on top of zucchini noodles for a decadent weeknight dinner!

Prep time: 10 minutes | Cooking Time: 35 minutes | Servings: 1

Ingredients
- 1/2 red pepper, diced
- 1 Tablespoon olive oil
- 1 teaspoon red pepper flakes
- 1/2 lemon, sliced into three equal sized medallions
- 1 6 oz fillet cod, preferably Ocean Safe certified wild caught
- 1 teaspoon dried oregano
- 1 teaspoon dried thyme
- 1 teaspoon salt
- 1 teaspoon pepper

Instructions
2. Preheat the oven to 375F. Toss the pepper with the olive oil and a pinch of salt, and transfer the mixture into an ovenproof baking dish.
3. Bake for 20 minutes, until soft. Transfer the roasted pepper to a blender or food processor, and puree until smooth. Next, lay the cod onto a baking sheet lined with parchment. Preheat oven to 350F.
4. Lay the lemon wheels onto a baking sheet lined with parchment, and place the fish on top. Season the fish with the salt, pepper, thyme, red pepper flakes and oregano, and spoon the pureed pepper over top.
5. Bake 12 minutes. Turn the broiler on to high, and broil for 5 minutes. Serve immediately.

Nutritional info per serving:
Calories 336 | Carbs 6 g | Fats 16.2 g | Proteins 40 g

Beef Stew

This stew is warm and hearty, and really yummy!

Prep time: 10 minutes | Cooking Time: 55 minutes | Servings: 4

Ingredients:
- 1 lb. flank steak, cut into chunks
- 1 Tablespoon olive oil
- 1 Tablespoon thyme
- 1 Tablespoon salt
- 4 cups beef stock
- 2 Tablespoons butter
- 1 carrot, chopped
- 2 stalks celery, chopped

- 1 14.5 oz can dice tomatoes
- 1/4 onion, chopped
- 2 cloves garlic, minced
- 2 Tablespoons Worcestershire sauce
- 1/2 cup red wine (optional)
- 1 cup heavy cream

Instructions:

1. Preheat a large pot over medium heat. Drizzle the oil, and brown the beef on all sides- about 4 minutes. Remove from pan and set aside.
2. In the same pot, melt in the butter and sauté the vegetables with the salt, until soft - about 3 minutes. Add in the herbs. Return the beef back to the pot.
3. Add the stock and Worcestershire sauce and wine. Bring to a boil, then reduce heat to low. Simmer 25 minutes. Stir in the cream, and simmer another 15 minutes. You could also make this in a crockpot!
4. After browning the beef, add the rest of the ingredients (except cream) to the crockpot and cook on low 4-6 hours.
5. Turn heat off, let sit for 30 minutes to cool down, then add the heavy cream.

Nutritional info per serving:
Calories 450 | Carbs 4.5 g | Fats 30.4 g | Proteins 35 g

Fish Tacos

Using leftover Baja Style Halibut Salad, you can easily make these fish tacos for a quick, easy cold lunch! Perfect for a hot day!

Prep time: 5 minutes | Cooking Time: 0 minutes | Servings: 3

Ingredients
- 1 serving Baja Style Halibut Salad
- 8 large pieces iceberg lettuce
- 2 Tablespoons salsa (optional)

Instructions

1. Flake the fish and mix with the salad. Lay out 1-2 pieces of lettuce to create a wrap, and spoon 1/4 of the mixture into the center.
2. Wrap to form a little taco. Continue until all ingredients have been used. Serve with salsa.

Nutritional info per serving:
Calories 740 | Carbs 7 g | Fats 40 g | Proteins 95 g

Appendix : Recipes Index

A

A Green Bean Mixture 44
Acorn Squash with Mango Chutney 39
Almond and Blistered Beans 46
Almond bread with a delicate crust 72
Almond Butter Fat Bombs 105
Almond Buttery Green Cabbage 38
Almond Cinnamon Beef Meatballs 55
Almond Joy 89
Almond Pumpkin Pudding 103
Apple bread with horseradish and pistachios 71
Apple Slices 37
Asian Beef Stew 55
Asian Pork Hock 57
Asparagus and Artichoke Salad 22
Avgolemono Soup 25
Avocado Fries 48
Avocado Gazpacho 77
Avocado Mug Bread 67
Avocado Shrimp Salad 59
Avocado Spring Rolls 51
Avo-Tacos 14

B

Baby Kale and Yogurt Smoothie 100
Baby Potatoes 40
Baked Brie 106
Baked Chicken Fajitas 52
Baked Chicken Wings 53
Baked Salmon 58
Banana Hazelnut Waffles 18
Barbecue Chicken Pizza Soup 25
Basil Tomato Frittata 63
Beef Casserole 54
Beef Muffins 78
Beef Roast 55
Beef Shawarma 58
Beef Stew 107
Berry Acai Smoothie 99
Blackberry Smoothie 99
Blueberry and Soy Smoothie 99
Blueberry Avocado Smoothie 99
Boston Baked Beans Candy 94
Bourbon Candy Balls 96
Breakfast Cheesy Sausage 12
Brittle Butterscotch Candy 95
Broccoli Crunchies 44
Broccoli salad with fresh dill 29
Broccoli Stir Fry 35
Brussels and Pistachios 38
Brussels's Fever 39
Buffalo Cashews 44
Bulgur bread 70
Butter Coffee 75
Butter Tossed Asparagus 103
Buttery Lamb Chops 56
Buttery Shrimp 59

C

Candy Dots 89
Caramelized Onion 43
Caramelized Onions 103
Cardamom-Cinnamon Spiced Coco-Latte 101
Cashew Sauce 37
Cashew Siam Salad 21
Cauliflower and Mushroom Risotto 45
Cauliflower Cakes 40
Cauliflower Curry Soup 51
Cauliflower Frittata 63
Cauliflower Mash 36
Cauliflower Rice 47
Cauliflower Soufflé 36
Cauliflower Toast with Avocado 12
Celery and Almond Butter 105
Cheddar Cauliflower Bites 79
Cheese Almond Pancakes 62
Cheese sausage bread 67
Cheesecake Bites 80
Cheesecake Pudding 90
Cheesy Fondue 104
Cheesy Spinach 34
Chia Seed Pudding 76
Chia Spinach Pancakes 63
Chicken Chili Soup 32
Chicken Lime Soup 31
Chicken with Spinach Broccoli 53
Chinese Bok Choy 33
Choco Milk Smoothie 100
Choco-Coco Milk Shake 99
Chocolate Avocado Pudding 103
Chocolate Bonbons 88
Chocolate Cake 85
Chocolate Chip Balls 80
Chocolate Chip Cookies 92
Chocolate Chip Waffles 12
Chocolate Coconut Bites 88
Chocolate Coconut Cookies 92
Chocolate Covered Almonds 89
Chocolate Fudge Bars 84
Chocolate-Coconut Shake 102

Cilantro and Leeks Dip 78
Cinnamon & Nutmeg Cake 86
Clementine and Pistachio Ricotta 13
Coconut and Cauliflower Rice with Chili 41
Coconut Bars 80
Coconut Cauliflower Rice 62
Coconut Chocolate Bars 84
Coconut Crepes 15
Coconut Lemon Custard Pie 91
Coconut milk bread 68
Coconut No-Bake Cookies 93
Coffee Cake 87
Cream & Berries Cake 87
Cream Cheese Cookies 93
Cream Cheese Spread 77
Cream Of Mushroom Soup 26
Cream Of Mushroom Soup 27
Cream Of Tomato Soup 27
Creamed Spinach with Cheese 34
Creamy Beef Stroganoff 56
Creamy Brussels Sprout 35
Creamy Choco Shake 100
Creamy Cinnamon Coffee 76
Creamy Wake-Me-Up Smoothie 102
Crispy Cookies 97
Crispy Kale 43
Crispy Tofu Burgers 52
Crystal Candy Skewers 95
Cumin bread 73
Curry Mayonnaise 104

D
Delicious Bacon Chicken 53
Delicious Garlic Tomatoes 37

E
Easy Cheesy Artichokes 33
Egg bread 68
Egg Crepes with Avocados 13
Egg Roll Bowl 18
English Custard 90

F
Fat-Bomb Frappuccino 20
Fennel Grill Pork Chops 57
Feta Kale Frittata 63
Fifth Avenue Candy 92
Fish Tacos 108
Fresh Breath Mints 94
Fried Apple 41
Frozen Yogurt 80
Fruity Morning Smoothie 102

G
Garbanzo and Spinach Beans 36
Garden Greens & Yogurt Shake 101
Garlic and Kale Platter 39
Garlic and Mushroom Crunch 41
German bread linz 71
Ginger and Orange "Beets" 40
Ginger Snap Cookies 93
Gingerbread-Spiced Breakfast Smoothie 15
Ginger-Spiced Coconut-Milk Shake 101
Granola Bars 85
Green Bean Fries 104
Green Bean Roast 45
Green Cabbage with Bacon 33
Green Tahini 104
Grilled Salmon 60

H
Ham and Cheese Pockets 13
Ham And Green Bean Soup 24
Hazelnut and Coconut Shake 101
Hazelnut honey bread 67
Hazelnut-Lettuce Yogurt Shake 100
Hazelnut-Mocha Shake 102
Herb Pork Roast 57
Herbs Spread 78
Honey and Coconut Porridge 39
Honey bread with cream and coconut milk 71

I
Iced Keto Coffee 74
Instant Pot Beans & Ham Soup 21
Italian blue cheese bread 71

J
Jalapeno Bacon Cheddar Soup 30
Jalapeno Pepper Soup 31
Japanese Cabbage Dish 38
Jicama Fries 74

K
Kale and Carrot with Tahini Dressing 42
Kale Muffins 77
Kelp noodle salad 22
Keto Avocado Toast 12
Keto bread rolls 65
Keto Breakfast Porridge 18
Keto Choco "Oats" 18
Keto coconut bread rolls 66
Keto Ice Cream Coffee mix 75
Keto Mocha 74
Keto Turkish Coffee 74
Key Lime Pie 81
Kidney Beans and Cilantro 43

L
- Lemon Bars 85
- Lemon Cheesecake Mousse 89
- Lemon Coconut Cake 82
- Lemon Herb Lamb Chops 56
- Lemony Sprouts 46
- Low carb bread rolls (without eggs) 66
- Low-Carb Breakfast "Couscous" 15
- Low-carb clover rolls 65
- Low-carb dinner rolls 65
- Low-carb fried kale and broccoli salad 29

M
- Maple Glazed Carrots 40
- Mashed Celeriac 37
- Matcha Avocado Pancakes 15
- Meat-Free Breakfast Chili 17
- Mexican Beef 54
- Mexican Beef with Zucchini 54
- Mexican Chicken 53
- Milk almond bread 72
- Mixed cabbage coleslaw 30
- Mixed Nuts Choco Candy Clusters 97
- Multi-grain bread 69
- Mushroom Zoodle Pasta 49

N
- No Bake Coconut Bars 83
- Nut Butter Cookies 93
- Nutty Arugula Yogurt Smoothie 100
- Nutty Choco Milk Shake 100
- Nutty Cookies 97

O
- Olive Cheese Omelet 62
- Orange Walnut Cookies 94
- Oriental red cabbage salad 28
- Overnight Oat Bowl 14

P
- Parmesan Meatballs 58
- Parmesan Salmon 61
- Parmesan Zucchini Chips 62
- Parsley Dip 77
- Peanut Brittle 94
- Peanut Butter Bars 83
- Pecan Brittle Squares 95
- Pecan Candies 96
- Pepper Jack Cauliflower 42
- Protein Muffins 64
- Pumpkin Cheesecake Mousse 90
- Pumpkin Spice Mug Cake 82

Q
- Quick Breakfast Yogurt 16
- Quick Veggie Protein Bowl 49

R
- Raspberry Chia Pudding 106
- Raspberry Chocolate Fudge 106
- Raspberry Ice Cream 81
- Red Pepper Cod 107
- Rice bread 72
- Rice bread with soy sauce 73
- Roasted Onions and Green Beans 45

S
- Salmon Patties 59
- Salmon with Sauce 60
- Salted Macadamias 105
- Sausage bread 67
- Seafood salad with avocado 30
- Shrimp and Broccoli 58
- Shrimp and Garlic 59
- Shrimp Bowls 78
- Shrimp Scampi 60
- Shrimp Stir Fry 61
- Simple keto bread 69
- Snickerdoodle Cookies 98
- Southern Salad 42
- Spaghetti Squash 41
- Spiced Tofu and Broccoli Scramble 17
- Spicy Cauliflower Soup 25
- Spicy Mayo 106
- Spicy Mushrooms 35
- Spicy Satay Tofu Salad 23
- Spinach & Cauliflower Soup 28
- Spinach Chips 77
- Strawberry Chia Pudding Popsicles 107
- Strawberry Coconut Shake 101
- Stuffed Zucchini 48
- Summertime Veggies 43
- Superfood Soup 24

T
- Tahini Sauce 105
- Tasty Chicken Egg Rolls 76
- Tasty Green Salad 22
- Thai Chicken Coconut Soup 23
- Thai Iced Tea 75
- The Asian Chickpea Pancake 14
- The Brussels Platter 42
- Thyme Leek Snack Bowls 78
- Tiramisu Chia Pudding 19
- Toast bread 70
- Tofu and Spinach Frittata 19
- Tofu Cheese Nuggets & Zucchini Fries 50
- Tomato Dip 79
- Tomato Platter 46
- Truffle Parmesan Salad 21

Tuna Salad 60
Turmeric Dip 79
Turnips Mashed 61

V

Vanilla Berry Mug Cake 81
Vanilla Custard 75
Vanilla Pana Cotta 75
Vegan Breakfast Biscuits 16
Vegan Breakfast Hash 19
Vegan Breakfast Muffins 16
Vegan Breakfast Sausages 16
Vegan Breakfast Skillet 19
Vegan Cream Of Broccoli Soup 26
Vegan Cream Of Broccoli Soup 27
Vegan Southwestern Breakfast 17
Vizza 49

W

Walnut bread 70
Warm Broccoli Salad Bowl 34

Y

Yellow-beet salad with anchovies 27
Yogurt Popsicles 81

Z

Zucchini Boats 45
Zucchini Eggplant with Cheese 61
Zucchini salad with eggs 29

www.ingramcontent.com/pod-product-compliance
Lightning Source LLC
Chambersburg PA
CBHW081117080526
44587CB00021B/3638